THE GAP

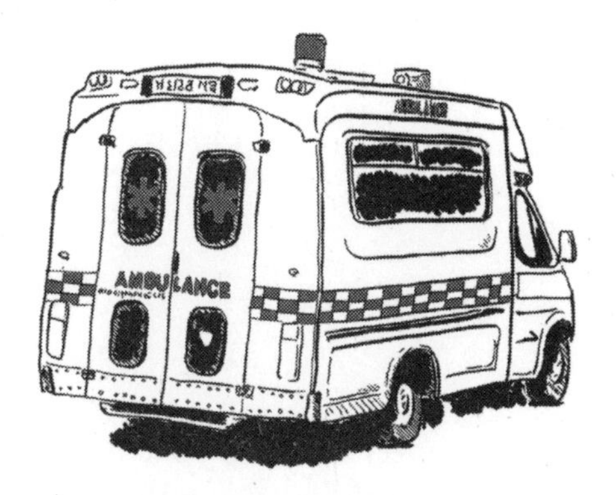

Benjamin Gilmour has been a paramedic for twenty-two years and holds a Bachelor of Paramedicine and a Master of Public Health. He is also an author, screenwriter and film director. His film *Jirga* was Australia's submission for Best Foreign Language Film Oscar, 2019, and the screenplay won the NSW Premier's Literary Award (Betty Roland Prize) for Screenwriting. He is the author of several books, including the bestselling *Paramedico: Around the World by Ambulance.* Benjamin is based in northern New South Wales, where he lives with his wife, Kaspia, and three children.

benjamingilmour.com

Also by Benjamin Gilmour:

Warrior Poets

Paramedico

The Travel Bug

Cameras & Kalashnikovs

BENJAMIN GILMOUR

THE GAP

VIKING
an imprint of
PENGUIN BOOKS

Pseudonyms have been used in this book and other details altered where necessary to protect the identity and privacy of people mentioned.

VIKING

UK | USA | Canada | Ireland | Australia
India | New Zealand | South Africa | China

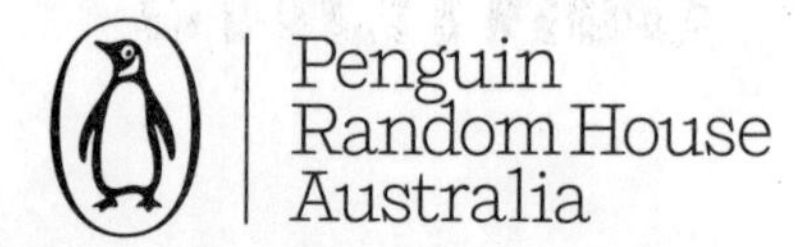

Viking is part of the Penguin Random House group of companies whose addresses can be found at global.penguinrandomhouse.com.

First published by Viking, an imprint of
Penguin Random House Australia Pty Ltd, 2019

Cover design and illustration by Alex Ross © Penguin Random House Australia Pty Ltd
Typeset in 13/19 pt Bembo by Midland Typesetters, Australia

Printed and bound in Australia by Griffin Press, part of Ovato, an accredited ISO AS/NZS 14001 Environmental Management Systems printer

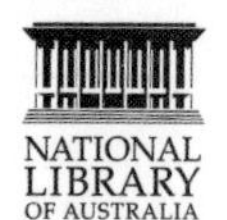

A catalogue record for this book is available from the National Library of Australia

ISBN 978 1 76089 020 9

penguin.com.au

CONTENTS

Author's Note	vii
Chapter 1	1
Chapter 2	17
Chapter 3	31
Chapter 4	43
Chapter 5	65
Chapter 6	81
Chapter 7	95
Chapter 8	113
Chapter 9	127
Chapter 10	147
Chapter 11	165
Chapter 12	181
Chapter 13	195

Chapter 14 213
Chapter 15 229
Chapter 16 251
Chapter 17 259
Chapter 18 271

AUTHOR'S NOTE

This book has been written from detailed notes I took while working as a paramedic on ambulances in Sydney during the summer of 2007–08. An early draft was finished in 2009, but I considered the material too sensitive to publish at the time. Ten years on, enough has changed to allow for the story to be told.

Although this book narrates true events, the names and ages of patients have been altered, as have locations, times and other identifying features, to protect their privacy. The names of my fellow paramedics have also been disguised, with the exception of my friend John, and in some cases the characteristics of two or more colleagues have intentionally been merged to further respect their wish for anonymity. For narrative purposes, there are instances where the order of some events has been shifted.

Conversations are either recorded word for word based on my notes, or roughly as I remember them.

All views expressed in this book are mine alone and do not represent those of other paramedics or my employer. Nor does my attitude and conduct in this book necessarily reflect the person and paramedic I am today, ten years later, or the attitude and conduct of my colleagues in the present. I no longer work in Sydney, and every main player in this book has moved on too. But what will never change is the trauma and death paramedics are exposed to, and the impact this can have on us and the way we manage our mental health.

While there are many external factors that affect paramedics' wellbeing beyond the influence of an employer, since writing this book a decade ago remarkable work has been done by ambulance services in Australia to address the emotional and psychological needs of staff. NSW Ambulance, for example, has hired full-time psychologists, expanded their chaplaincy and peer support programs and conducted wellness workshops. While organisational change can be complex and slow, the shift in workplace culture and the generous funding and strategies implemented to improve paramedic wellbeing should be acknowledged.

A word of warning: there are moments of black comedy in this book that some readers may find confronting. But an authentic narrative of this kind cannot exist without the gallows humour that paramedics are famous for, a humour shared by many doctors and nurses, police and undertakers.

Studies have shown that this type of humour has an important psychological and social function in professions that deal with pain and sorrow on a daily basis. It's a way of slaying the monster, of dealing with stress and keeping up morale.

There is also frank discussion of mental illness and suicide. The manuscript has been assessed by psychologists at Everymind for impact on vulnerable readers, and dozens of changes have been made to soften imagery and remove explicit detail. Even so, if you feel triggered while reading, please reach out, make a call and ask for help. A list of excellent crisis support services that can assist you are included in the back of the book.

Lastly, since writing about some of my experiences with poor survival rates of cardiac arrest, I've been involved in more than half a dozen saves. Increased community CPR and access to defibrillators, along with improved paramedic resuscitation techniques, have played a part in this.

Special thanks goes to my former colleagues, both paramedics and nurses, for their ongoing friendship and reading of the manuscript; to my brilliant publisher Sophie Ambrose, editor Tom Langshaw and agent James Wills; to psychologist Sara Bartlett and the suicide prevention team at Everymind; to the Dixon family, Antony Loewenstein, John Zubrzycki, Tony Ayres, Craig Henderson, Marele Day and Alex Warner; and to my parents and my ever-supportive wife, Kaspia.

Benjamin Gilmour
August 2019

CHAPTER 1

At the highest point of The Gap, where the clifftop rises like a tower, it is ninety metres to the sea. Tourists and daytrippers come in groups to stand at the wood-and-wire fence, inhaling the sunrise. They chatter about nothing of consequence, but are quickly made speechless by nature's might. I've seen them stand like people at a crossroads, suddenly conscious of their smallness. The Gap is a place of great change, new journeys, different paths. But for others who come, their hope is long lost. To them, The Gap is a backdrop for the final act of life. It's the edge of the world from which they leave. Fifty or more go over each year, from the top, or further around where the fence is easier to scale. They do it at dawn, in the heaviest rain, and on the quietest of nights.

For us local paramedics the beauty up here is hard to admire.

We're called to a woman in her twenties who's been seen climbing the fence. I slow the ambulance and turn around, head back that way.

'How inconsiderate,' says John, my paramedic partner. 'Killing herself so close to our knock-off time.'

He's the king of dark humour, our John. It diffuses frustrations, lightens a little the tragedies we see, and helps us to get through each shift.

'Least we've come well prepared.' John opens the glovebox and pulls out a packet of peanuts.

'Ever nibbled Nobby's Nuts?'

Standing by at suicide attempts can lead to awful hunger. Some suicidal patients will hesitate for hours. For paramedics the tedium of the wait is bad enough, but the hunger is worse. Emergency nuts have long been the answer.

Patients who are still on the edge when we get to the scene don't often follow through. Many others have fallen before we manage to get there. Sometimes we see their bodies on the rocks or in the water. If the chopper or rescue squad don't reach them in time, they can disappear forever.

Just past the little row of shops at Watsons Bay a police officer waves us down. He approaches and says the girl can't be found. He thinks she must have gone over. Her sneakers were neatly placed at the edge. Why people leave their shoes is anyone's guess. Perhaps to not drag any dirt from this world into the next.

We park the ambulance behind the girl's blue hatchback and see a man – must be her father – cross the road. John opens the bag of salted peanuts, throws a few into his mouth. He crunches down, then passes the packet over.

We watch the father and the police officer through the windscreen. It's like a silent movie. All I hear is our crinkling peanut packet and the crunching of Nobby's Nuts as the tragedy unfolds.

A constable extends his baton with a flick. He smashes the driver's window of the girl's car and carefully reaches in, taking a folded letter off the dash. He hands it to the father. With trembling fingers the man slowly opens it. As he reads his daughter's suicide note his lips begin to quiver. He runs a hand through his thinning hair: once, twice, a third time. Then he finishes reading and his chest begins to heave in sighs of grief. His head tilts back and he closes his eyes like somebody injured. When he opens them again a gush of tears spills down his face. We're mesmerised by his anguish, his agony.

'Fuck it,' says John, twisting the top of the packet and returning it to the glovebox. He gets out and walks to the back of the wagon to get the father a blanket. Then he goes and puts it round the man's shoulders. It's summertime, and not even cold. But the man huddles into it like a child. John puts a comforting hand on his shoulder, stands beside him in silence.

Easing pain is our job. It's natural to want to reassure this father, perhaps remind him that his daughter isn't alone, that she's with a thousand souls who've gone before her. But John knows, as I do, that the man has lost his little girl and no words can bring her back. She can never be a number, never like the rest who've ended their lives up here. She's the world to him, the centre of the world, the one he might have saved. The one *we* might have saved, if we'd reached her in time.

We streak into the city on another urgent call. An old man on Victoria Street, Kings Cross, hasn't been seen for days. Usually it's a case of someone going on holiday without informing their neighbours. But every now and then we find a dead body.

The neighbour meets us at the entrance, says, 'The guy, his name is Stanley, he's an artist type.'

We knock at the door, but don't hear an answer.

'You boot, I'll shoulder,' says John, looking over.

When the door splinters open we find Stanley on the floor, conscious and a bit confused, mumbling and muttering. There's weakness down his left side and his speech is slightly slurred, and whenever he opens his mouth we see his tongue has gone purple.

'Ever seen that in a stroke?' I ask John.

'Been eating crayons,' John speculates. He puts a finger into Stanley's mouth and pulls out a stick of lilac.

'There you go,' John says with pride.

As we carry Stanley out we see portraits on the walls, all of the same young woman nude. In one framed work her breasts are resting on her belly like two small cupcakes, and her slightly parted legs show a hint of pubic hair.

'You've got a muse?' John asks him.

The old man's face lights up, his confusion gone.

'That's Helena,' he says, now smiling.

Back in the seventies Helena used to 'work the street' in front of his block, he tells us. Between her clients she'd come to his place to have a rest. He'd serve her Bushells tea and Anzac biscuits, and she'd sit for him. He'd sketch Helena almost every day. Soon enough she was the only subject he was interested in. He sketched her several times a week for years. And then one day she vanished.

'No goodbyes, no nothing,' Stanley says. 'I knew she'd disappear eventually.'

We lift him up and take him to the ambulance. He'll need a brain scan to check for a stroke.

'That's why I drew Helena as much as I could, why I still draw her now, why I copy my portraits over and over, so I'll never forget, and her face and her body will be fresh in my mind. That's love, I suppose. She's been gone thirty years; she could've died long ago for all I know. But even if she's dead, she lives on in my heart.'

At the hospital later I ask John if he's ever had a muse. My girlfriend Kaspia, with her classic Renaissance figure, is the perfect muse for me.

'Antonio? A muse?' John laughs, referring to his long-time Brazilian boyfriend. 'He's got a good body, but I wouldn't sit there sketching it. Not like you, sketching everything in your little black book.'

So he still has a problem with my little black book. It's a Moleskine diary I occasionally write in, full of drawings of faces, snippets of dialogue, the stuff anyone interested in observing and writing makes note of.

'When you first arrived at Bondi everyone thought you were spying.'

'Spying? Who for – the Russians?'

'Bugger the Russians,' he says. 'Ambulance management more like. We thought you were gathering evidence on *us*, your fellow paramedics, passing it on, up the bloody chain.'

I could tell at the time my colleagues at Bondi were nervous. It didn't help that I'd stumbled on their secret brewery set-up in an unused laundry of the ambulance station. At first I'd mistaken it for a meth lab. I mentioned my discovery to John, and it vanished overnight.

'You can't have been that worried,' I say to John. 'You've been telling me your scandalous stories from the day we met.'

John laughs. 'Yeah, probably.'

'Yeah, for sure,' I reply. It's always when I'm obviously jotting away in my little black book that John will share his most salacious tales of life as a handsome gay man in Sydney, about ambulance work in the eighties, about smoking on the way to emergencies and the triple-0 discos, the burnouts in vacant lots and happy gas on night shifts. Never once has he held up his hand to stop me transcribing his stories. Never once has he asked me to omit a sordid detail.

'Anyway, I'm not always writing about you,' I tell him.

He's suddenly offended. 'Why not? Don't tell me I'm boring.'

But he knows he isn't boring. He's never been boring.

They say the dead are the only ones John can't make laugh. Although I'm sure I've seen a few of them smile.

On a Kings Cross street corner an alcoholic we know is lying on his back. A crowd stands around him, gawking. Like many people with alcohol addictions who try to stop their drinking, Bobby will throw the occasional fit.

We discuss the best way to get him to our stretcher. He's breathing okay; just a bit groggy. As we're moving to lift him a man in a suit taps me on the shoulder and says, 'Excuse me, don't you think you should put him in the recovery position?'

'Pardon?' I reply, taken aback.

'Recovery position. I did a first-aid course and that's what I'd do if I were you.'

John chuckles beside me. 'Be our guest, sir,' he says, lowering Bobby.

We step back a little to allow the man in. The good Samaritan hesitates, then with annoyance he sets down his briefcase and kneels by the patient. His lips curl in disgust at Bobby's unwashed T-shirt and grimy black jeans. Then he places his clean office hands on our patient's leg and shoulder. I'm surprised and impressed. But just as the corporate guy rolls Bobby over, our patient wakes up and opens his eyes.

'What tha fuck are you doing?' Bobby yells in anger. 'Get tha fuck off me! Leave me alone or I'll kill ya!' He spits and kicks a leg at the stranger.

'Careful,' John warns.

The businessman stumbles backwards in horror. John steadies his elbow to stop him from falling. Then the man grabs his briefcase and hurries away.

Yeah, John's never boring. Maybe it's why he's mentioned so often in my little black book.

Bobby snores on our trolley in the emergency-department corridor of St Vincent's Hospital, waiting for a bed. This wait can sometimes take a while, so John has made us tea and sits beside Bobby slurping his loudly. *Slurp, snore, slurp, snore.* The noise gets the attention of a few passing nurses, who laugh and shake their heads at my partner. John takes things seriously when he needs to. But between those fleeting moments, the job is a circus.

Ten minutes later we're rushing to an asthma attack in Bondi Junction. Our control centre has taken a call from a woman too breathless to pass on her address. Luckily it's come from a landline, and the call has been traced.

Shooting through a red light, I'm careful not to spill John's hospital tea in his lap. 'Don't you scald my greatest asset!' he warns me.

The caller doesn't answer the doorbell when we ring. We knock and shout and ring again. Nothing. We see the curtains drawn and speculate that the woman must have made her own way to hospital. Perhaps her husband or a friend has picked her up, John says. There's no car out front, and when I look through the mail slot there's no movement in the house.

'No one's home,' I say.

John returns to the ambulance to finish his tea.

'Take a look round the back,' he calls over his shoulder.

I head down the alleyway alongside the house and find the rear entrance. There's a shabby wall too high to see over, and a wooden gate that's locked. I grab the top of the brickwork and try my best to scale the wall, then curse as the soles of my rescue boots struggle to get purchase. But I make it over, and then I'm down the other side. Few professions allow a person to break and enter like this, and we've done it twice today already. It's rather enjoyable, a bit James Bond, although usually there's no one home. Once, in North Sydney, I climbed a drainpipe to a balcony and into a flat where I found a woman murdered in a gruesome crime of passion. Now and then we'll get a case like that.

'Hello?' I call out.

There's a sliding door to the sunroom. I knock. No response. Cupping my hands around my face, I peer into the gloom. It takes a few seconds for my eyes to adjust. When they do, I see indoor palms, some hanging ferns . . . and a pair of skinny legs sticking out from behind a bamboo lounge. I squint again. Definitely a pair of skinny legs.

'Damn it,' I say.

I whisk the portable radio from my waist and call for backup, hoping John will hear my transmission and bring our gear to the front door. Then I dash round the side of the house and find a tiny bathroom window slightly open. There's a rusty barbecue nearby so I roll it against the wall and clamber up. I push the window up and go in feet first. There's hardly enough room to squeeze through, but I've had plenty of practice. In my second year as an ambo a few of my colleagues saw me on the dance floor and began to call me Snake Hips. Ever since then I've been the one they send through cat flaps.

There's a bang and a clatter as I knock a mug of toothbrushes onto the tiles. Then my feet hit the ground.

When I reach the woman in the sunroom I see she's blue in the face. First I go to the front door and unlock it for John. I'm relieved to see him waiting there with our oxygen, defibrillator and drug kit.

'I nearly choked on my tea,' he says, pushing into the hall and handing me a bag.

The woman lies on her back, still clutching her phone. She's got no pulse so I start CPR. Under my hand I feel a few ribs pop off the sternum. Meanwhile, John cuts off her singlet and connects the defibrillator. She's in ventricular fibrillation, a quivering of the heart. We push some buttons and the machine charges with a whine. It's an ear-piercing sound, rising in pitch like an air-raid siren. With it rises the tension in the room, as if a bomb is about to go off.

'Press to shock,' comes the robotic voice prompt.

John calls 'Clear!' and checks that I don't have a hand on the patient. Then he presses the shock button and the woman jolts with the current.

Her heart flatlines.

Our backup crew comes through the door and prepares to intubate while John cannulates for adrenalin. Then, a minute later, the woman's husband arrives home, whistling and swinging his satchel. It's just like any other day. Only this time he stumbles in on four paramedics trying to revive his lifeless wife, who lies there with her bra cut off.

'Sorry, mate,' I say. 'But she called us and we found her not breathing. There's no pulse. You don't have to look if you don't want to.' I tell him this while pumping on her chest.

The man is rooted to the spot, snap-frozen. When I glance his way again, he seems to have taken my advice. Oddly, though, he's now sitting on the lounge blankly watching a soap on television, cigarette between his fingers. John notices too, and raises an eyebrow. Smoke creeps around the room like a ghost. Immediate reactions to traumatic stress can be unpredictable, bizarre even; we accept that. Some people scream, some laugh, some run. Others smoke and watch daytime TV. Reactions to death can make as much sense as the death itself. The same could be said, I guess, about the paramedic's black humour.

At Prince of Wales Hospital, after more resuscitation, the woman is pronounced dead. This doesn't surprise me; it never does. People think saving lives is our bread and butter. But a full recovery after cardiac arrest is the rarest of things.

John's ready to go again, and so am I. We hope our next case will be less of a downer. But our job is a lucky dip of drama; we never know what's coming.

The billionaire's wife has lips like a groper's. They open and close and splutter through tears. Her name is Felicity and her wedding ring, with its giant diamond set in gold, is abandoned on the table. She's alone in her mansion as the sun drops down behind a view of the harbour.

'How can we help you, Felicity?' asks John, sinking into a leather recliner like he lives here too. He knows how to make himself comfortable, John. Whatever the case, he'll breeze in and, unless it's a hoarder's home, go straight for the sofa. There he'll do what few men can; cross his legs and his arms at the same time, before casually getting a history from the patient as if he's at a cocktail party.

'Please help . . . I nearly killed myself.'

'Nearly?'

'Yes. At the last minute I stopped myself.'

'You stayed your own hand.'

'I did.'

'You saved your own life.'

'Yes.'

'Good. So what are we here for?'

'It might happen again.'

'You've been feeling depressed?'

'Fucking depressed.'

'If you're suicidal we need to take you to hospital.'

'I hate him! I hate him!'

'Who do you hate?

'Jeremy.'

'Your husband?'

She nods. 'The bastard. He can't do this anymore. He's got me in a snow dome and he's shaking me up. He's always off on business, out of town, overseas. All to make me happy, so he says. Times are tough. Works late, every night. And what do I do? Sit here alone, snorting cocaine. And tomorrow, what then? Go to the races on my own. Imagine, the races on your own!'

Felicity's case isn't unusual. Sometimes, in the pursuit of money, other things are neglected, important things like health, spirituality and love. It's no wonder the most affluent can be the most miserable. My work in the eastern suburbs has proven this to me. Anxiety, depression and suicide rates are out of control. Just yesterday we counselled a chief executive who could 'only' sell his company for $25 million. He too had lost the will to live.

'On paramedic wages, with less to lose, we'll never have these problems,' says John.

As we drive back to the station we stop at a liquor store to pick up a six-pack. We often have beers together after work; it's our way of debriefing. But we shouldn't buy booze in uniform; it's not allowed. When I say this to John he fixes me with a look and says, 'Who're you working for? Us or them? Don't be a killjoy. No one gives a shit.'

When he returns to the ambulance he tells me a man waiting in the queue at the bottle shop tapped him on the shoulder and thanked him for saving his life last year. The guy then insisted on paying for John's beer.

'And there you were worrying about complaints,' John says. 'Truth is, everyone in this country wants to shout us a drink.'

I ask John for the story, the life-saving deed he performed on his benefactor.

John shrugs. 'Who bloody knows. I've never seen him before. He probably mistook me for another ambo. But I'll always take credit for saving a life. Wouldn't you?'

CHAPTER 2

Beams of light sneak between the shutters as I sleep through my snooze alarms. I've woken alone again in the apartment I rent on the top floor of a Darlinghurst terrace. I think about Kaspia, my girlfriend and muse, my travel companion, a burlesque dancer, the woman I love, who is no longer here.

It's a trial separation, we agreed, for three months. We're in love but we fight way too much. It's hard to understand, most of all for us. A decade of travelling and living together, and now this. Separation. Kaspia in a place in Balmain, me here in Darlinghurst. We haven't talked for weeks and I'm not as relieved as I thought I would be. My apartment's too quiet, too empty, too dark. And the only arguments are down on the street, between working girls and pimps. It's funny how they make me feel, these late-night shouting matches peppered with expletives. I get warm all over, nostalgic, and I'm reminded of the counsellor who told us once that arguments between couples are a special kind of intimacy.

I roll out of bed for a shower, then pull on my uniform. I turn on the hairdryer, comb up my quiff, add some wax. Half the job's done simply by having a smart presentation, winning the confidence of patients. It's reassuring to people. No matter how I feel or where I go, my comb comes along.

Like a seagull suspended by an updraught, the rescue chopper hovers over Bondi's northern cliffs and winches up a dead man.

We park the ambulance on the ninth hole of the golf course overlooking the sea. People are playing the eighth hole as the helicopter lands on the seventh to give us the body. It could be a fisherman swept off the rocks. But we suspect it's more likely a man who fell from The Gap last night. The outgoing crew told us about it. That's two gone over in a day and a half.

John looks at the golfers. 'You go to the trouble of killing yourself and no one seems to care. They just keep on hitting little balls into holes.'

The ambulance smells like fish and sea water on our drive

to the morgue. We stop to pick up coffee and croissants. There's bossa nova playing on the ambulance stereo.

The perils of the ocean are part of summer in this city. A bluebottle sting at Bronte Beach takes us back into our area, a catchment extending from Bronte to Point Piper and up to Watsons Bay. Swimming into a school of bluebottles can make a person rather sick, but this sting's not too bad. After treating and releasing the patient, John suggests we park the ambulance at the northern end of the beach. He's supposed to be doing his paperwork but instead he sits there gazing at one of the mansions the way a kid might look at a lolly shop. The multistorey building overlooking the ocean has heavily tinted windows for privacy. Everyone knows it's the house of Australian actor Heath Ledger.

'Did I ever tell you how much I love him?' says John.

'Yes, you did,' I reply.

John is a celebrity-watcher par excellence. At the hospital he browses the trashy magazines the nurses bring in, getting all the latest Hollywood gossip. Right now he's hoping Ledger will emerge on one of his balconies wearing nothing more than a bathrobe. Several months ago John was working with Jerry, another Bondi paramedic, when they saw Heath Ledger jogging between Bondi and Tamarama. As Jerry recounted it, John leant out the window of the ambulance and shouted,

'Yoo-hoo, Heath! Hello!' and gave the actor a big flamboyant wave. Apparently Ledger looked up, but didn't respond. No wave, no smile, nothing. He even seemed annoyed. The actor's response hurt John badly. He wouldn't let it go. Put him in a foul mood for weeks.

John opens the door of the ambulance and gets out. He smooths down the creases in his shirt with his hands.

'What're you doing?' I ask.

'Going up.'

'Up where?'

'To Heath's house.'

'What?'

He slams the door and starts climbing the stairs of the property. I wind down my window and call after him.

'John! Are you crazy?'

But he ignores me and keeps ascending the path to the mansion. Then he disappears around the side of the house. His derring-do is well known, but this could be going too far.

Five minutes tick by as I sit and imagine what trouble is brewing. Then I see John emerge and descend the path, hands in his pockets. He gets into the ambulance.

'Well?' I ask him.

He sighs. 'It was just his fucking PA again. When the guy opened the door I told him someone had called an ambulance and I needed to confirm with the actual resident personally if he or she needed help or not.'

'And?'

'Told me it was probably another prank call. Said Heath was perfectly okay. Then he closed the door in my face. Just like that. Can you believe it? Closed the door on a paramedic, a *respected* paramedic. I suppose it's how he's become after hassles with paparazzi.'

Paparazzi *and* paramedics, I'm tempted to say.

'You've got a boyfriend,' I remind him. 'Remember?'

John sighs and looks out the window. My comment ruins the atmosphere. We respond to a job in the city and John doesn't say a word on our drive to the scene.

Not far from the fountain in Hyde Park, a man in a beige suit approaches us. He points to a dishevelled woman on a bench and says, 'I was having my sandwich and that woman over there told me she was in pain, so I called you.'

When we get to her she hands John a scrap of paper, a handwritten note.

'What's this?' asks John.

'My shopping list,' she says.

'And?'

'My knees are giving me trouble. Can you drive me to Coles? The supermarket? I need to get my vitamins and garlic tablets from the chemist on the way, if that's okay.'

John stands like a statue, expressionless for a moment, the

shopping list fluttering between his finger and thumb. But the woman is up and already shuffling towards the ambulance. She has every intention of getting into it until I gently divert her to the nearest taxi stand.

'Listen,' I say once John and I are back in the ambulance, 'if Heath Ledger had actually *met* you, like *properly* met you, his PA might've let you in. So don't feel jilted. He hasn't had the pleasure of meeting you properly, that's all.'

John's about to reply when another man comes to the side of the ambulance and taps on the driver's window.

'Oh, God,' says John. 'Look at this guy. Our job was hard enough with *one* good Samaritan; now everyone's in on it. Fucking ridiculous.'

John winds down his window and says, 'No, sorry, we can't take you shopping, sir.'

The man is understandably confused for a second, then says, 'Righto, yes, no problem. Thing is, I just wanted to tell you there's a girl lying down over there near the giant chess-board. She says she feels sick.'

'Thanks very much,' says John, winding up the window. He hesitates for a moment, then puts the ambulance in reverse to take us out of the park.

'Come on, mate,' I say. 'We gotta check it out. We can't pretend –'

'Can't we?' he says. But he catches sight of the good

Samaritan glaring at us from the fountain. John puts his foot on the brake and lets out a long sigh. 'Bloody do-gooders,' he says, moving off in the direction of the patient.

Her name is Tammy; she's wearing a random assortment of clothing and she has a silver lip ring. John asks her how we can help and she asks for a lift to Sydney Hospital because she's 'spent the whole night drinking riesling'. She holds up a drained bag of cask wine.

'They took me up there yesterday too,' she adds.

The hospital in question is less than a hundred metres away, a short walk. But we're not in the mood for arguing; we just want to leave the park. So we offer Tammy a ride.

She tells us her dad used to be the only paramedic in a remote outback town.

'I don't speak to him anymore, he never cared for me, never hugged me. He was a druid and my mum was a witch, and a prostitute. They were in a secret coven in the bush and did this ceremony one night when the seasons changed. The coven decided my mum and dad should have a union, know what I mean. The two of them didn't even like each other. That's how I was born.'

While taking Tammy's blood pressure, John asks her how she ended up sleeping rough in the big bad city.

'I'm looking for a home,' she says.

After showing Tammy to a hospital bed she takes out a PlayStation Portable and starts to play.

'You have a PlayStation?' John points out, surprised.

'Yeah. It's pretty boring being homeless, you know,' she says without looking up.

John shakes his head. He probably thinks she's lazy. But I feel a special sympathy for this girl who was let down so terribly by one of our own troubled souls.

Our controller asks us to stand by in the city for a while. I turn down past the barracks towards George Street as I want to drive by the Strand Arcade, where Kaspia works her day job managing Love & Hatred, a jewellery boutique. I hope as I pass the entrance that she might emerge on her way to have lunch or to pop into Haigh's for some chocolate buttons. Just a short time ago, when we were living together in Bronte, she'd bring me home a little bag of buttons once a week. We'd go to the beach and sit on the sand and eat them together, looking at the sea.

But she's not walking out of The Strand and she's not in the queue for chocolate and my heart sinks low. I don't tell John. I just keep driving, regretting the day I agreed to her suggestion that we needed a break.

⋆

Ocean Street, which runs from Edgecliff Station to Centennial Park, is a corridor of green, the afternoon sun shimmering through its enormous overhanging trees. I cross double lines and watch a dozen cars veer away as I barrel down.

We park in the shadow of a blond-brick apartment block and lug our gear up the stairs to the fifth floor, where a man is experiencing chest pains. I'm surprised to see our sixty-four-year-old patient has three children under eight. They stand around him, stroking his arms and asking, 'What's wrong with Daddy? What's wrong with him?'

We suspect the man is having a heart attack and we're reluctant to let him walk. His face is ashen and sweat pours out in buckets. We give him aspirin and some other medication and quickly insert an IV. We've called a backup crew to help us carry him down, but they're taking too long. I hear them on the radio asking for an 'address check' and assume they're lost.

John and I decide not to wait any longer. We lift the man down ten flights of stairs, two between each floor, struggling with our oxygen pack and monitor. He's heavy and the stairwell is dangerously tight. The children follow behind, carrying the rest of our gear. Slightly flustered and puffed, I climb into the back of the ambulance as the man's wife, a woman in her mid-forties, arrives on the scene and catches my sleeve. Her eyes are desperate.

'Please save him,' she begs. 'He's got three kids, look at them . . .' She points at the children, who stand bewildered at the roadside. I pause for a moment to glance at them, then acknowledge her comment with a nod.

'Let's move,' I say to John with urgency.

Halfway to hospital the man begins to gasp, 'Can't breathe! Can't breathe!'

His wife's voice echoes in my head.

Please save him, he's got three kids, look at them . . .

I tell John to pick up speed. I rarely ask my partner to step on it like this. But he knows as I do that time is running out. John activates the siren to cross William Street, and a minute later we're at St Vincent's. We hand the patient over to the doctors and nurses, relieved he's survived his ride.

Three hours later, back at the emergency department with another case, we discover the man has passed away. A massive heart attack, a myocardial infarction. Too much of his heart muscle had died. His heart was useless; there was nothing they could do.

Please save him, he's got three kids . . . There at the roadside, before we left the scene, was the last time his wife and children saw him alive. John and I go quiet for a moment as the news sinks in. I suppose John's doing what I am: rewinding the case in his mind, playing it again, imagining how we might've done it better. What if we'd arrived a little earlier? What if we hadn't waited so long for backup to help us carry him out? Thoughts like this are torture, the line between self-assessment and self-blame tissue-thin.

'Let's not beat ourselves up,' says John. 'It's not our fault. He was having a heart attack. Big man, no elevator, narrow staircase. We did our best; we did what we could. His time was up.' John says the things we say to one another to stay afloat. It doesn't matter if they're true or not. To survive in this job we need to stave off the guilt with every worn-out platitude. He knows how badly I take these things. Maybe I'm softer than he is. Or perhaps I'm not as lenient on myself, not as ready as John is to shrug off the loss.

Before we go home for the day John looks me in the eye and says, 'Tell me truly, when was the last time you had a save? When was the last time you were a *hundred per cent sure* it was *you* and *only you* who tipped the balance?'

It doesn't take me long to answer. Twelve years as an ambo and not a single patient of mine whose heart has stopped has made it out of hospital alive. As far as I know, that is. I've helped save patients who weren't breathing: some moribund asthmatics and many heroin ODs. But turning around a cardiac arrest, a patient without a pulse, has eluded me.

My failure hangs like a cloud over every emergency call. Paramedics meet death on a regular basis and most of the time they can't do anything about it. Knowing that survival rates from cardiac arrest are grim doesn't assuage my guilt. Most of my colleagues have saved a few lives, and they have stories that keep them going. But not me. My confidence is shredded and I question my future.

Worse still is letting down the long line of life-savers I'm descended from. On my father's side there was a skilled pharmacist in the Victorian town of Craigieburn, who kept the notorious bushranger Ned Kelly alive on several occasions after firefights with police. The outlaw didn't dare visit a hospital for fear of getting arrested. My mother's German grandfather was a well-known fire chief in the heavily bombed city of Mönchengladbach during World War II, racing from one burning building to another, hauling women and children to safety, and picking up hundreds of bodies. My oma still has a black-and-white photo of him holding the nozzle of a fire hose like a trophy. Eventually he got dementia and ended up in a nursing home yelling 'Fire! Fire!' at random which, apparently, led to several evacuations his first week there. Then there was my Opa Willie, responsible for saving a boy who drowned in the Rhine River just after the war ended. His friend Fuss was swept off a sandbank and vanished. After searching frantically, my grandfather saw a scruff of ginger hair underwater and grabbed it, dragging out the lifeless boy. Without training or knowledge, seemingly from instinct, Willie cleared water from the boy's airway and moved his arms up and down above his head until Fuss heaved and spluttered and opened his eyes.

These were my forebears, their stories handed down to me as a child. Saving lives was in my blood, or it should have been.

'There's nothing you can do,' says John. 'Death's in our stars. It can't be tricked.'

But it *can* be delayed. Others have proven it. And we're employed to give it a shot.

Despite his pessimism, John seems in better spirits than earlier in the day. It's often the way; when he's down, I'm up. And when I'm down, he's up. I suppose it's an equilibrium that helps us to carry on with what we have to do, working against the odds.

CHAPTER 3

A new life entering the world is a soothing antidote to our business of death. It can be a messy affair, but the joy on the face of a parent when I hand them a newborn keeps me going in the more gruelling moments of the job. John, on the other hand, would be happiest never doing a childbirth again. He says he has no interest in vaginas. They're not his thing.

And so our Friday night begins with a delivery on the toilet.

'Done many?' asks John as we near the address.

'Plenty,' I reply.

'All yours then,' he says, half-smiling.

The emergency childbirths I've attended have been unforgettable. An unexpected breach, where I wondered for a while if the mother might be giving birth to an alien with a face like a bottom; a fifteen-year-old girl living with her parents, who'd hidden her pregnancy from them right until her waters broke on the kitchen floor; a pregnant woman calmly walking to the ambulance before climbing onto the stretcher and giving birth to her ninth child, which slid right out in a single push.

The front door of the ground-floor unit is open. John follows me down a dim and musty hallway towards high-pitched screaming. In a narrow bathroom at the end of the hall we see a woman lathered in sweat, squatting over her toilet with a baby's head between her legs. It's only taken a minute to respond to the call and arrive on scene, but the baby's face is an aubergine purple. Seconds count in situations like these, and I crouch down under the mother to support her newborn's head and check for a cord around its neck. There's nothing. I'm relieved.

'You're doing well,' I tell her. 'But you'll need to give a little push now. We need your baby out.'

She strains and grunts and curses, and it's lucky I have a good grip on the infant because it shoots into my hands like a cannonball. It's a relief when it happens so quickly, but much to my dismay there's half a litre of amniotic fluid backed up, which gushes out and drenches me from head to toe. Behind me a short giggle escapes from John, who's been watching all this from a comfortable distance. It doesn't matter. In my hands I'm holding a pink, living baby.

At least, I think I am. My vision is blurred by the amniotic fluid in my eyes and I don't have a free hand to wipe it off. When I try to speak more fluid runs from my hair into my mouth, and all I can manage is a helpless splutter. It's an unpleasant sour taste, this fluid, a little salty too. I spit a few times into the bathtub, then say to the woman, 'Congratulations, it's a boy.'

The woman takes her baby and cries with happiness.

'See?' whispers John as we help the mother and child to the ambulance. 'Dangerous things, vaginas. I'll never get that close to one.'

Not long after the job, on the way to pick up dinner, John says, 'Do you ever feel sorry for them?'

'Who?'

'The babies, coming into this fucked-up world.'

'Occasionally, I suppose.'

Now and then I'll look at parents and their environment, and I'll imagine the baby's life ahead. How can anyone *not* after seeing a heavily pregnant heroin user still working the streets, as we did last week? But then I remind myself that having a child can heal and transform a person. I hope it heals and transforms me one day.

★

School's out for the year and don't we know it. From 10 pm, drunk teenagers drop all over the place. They go hard too early, and always fall first.

A fifteen-year-old has been abandoned in a park by her friends. At least they called an ambulance before they fled.

'Pretty slack to leave a sick friend,' I say to John, as we load her up.

'You never did that?'

'Never.'

'Nor would my sisters' kids,' says John. They live up the coast and I often hear him speaking to them on the phone with enormous affection, as if they were his own.

A little later we find another girl lying in vomit in the well-heeled suburb of Dover Heights. She doesn't flinch when I take a pink iPhone from her jeans. I find 'Mum' in her contacts and dial the number. When her mother picks up I hear a rowdy dinner party going on in the background. The woman is slurring her words and doesn't sound sober enough to drive. But she says she'll come to meet us.

One of the girl's ugg boots has rolled into the gutter and is drenched in spew. John fishes it out with gloved fingers and brushes it down, looking disgusted.

'It's only vomit,' I say.

'It's a fucking *ugg boot*. The things we have to do in this thankless profession,' he grumbles, shoving the offending fashion item back on our patient's foot.

A group of curious bystanders has formed, and I ask a girl for a hair elastic. I gather our patient's golden locks from her pool of regurgitated pizza and make a bun of it.

When the mother turns up we help her daughter into the back seat of the family Mercedes. I make sure she's lying on her side for the short trip home.

There must have been another underage party nearby because our controller sends us to a third girl found lying in the bushes further down the road. She's conscious enough to tell us she sculled 'a drink that looks like water'. She's only fourteen, and this time we can't get through to her parents. We cart her off to the Children's Hospital in Randwick, where she can sober up. It's bizarre pushing intoxicated patients into paediatric hospitals full of crying babies and toddlers with temperatures. The age of sixteen is the cut-off, but I've come across overdose victims as young as twelve. As we roll through the doors we watch protective mothers reach out to shield their infants. The impulse is understandable. Intoxicated fourteen-year-olds can be as loud and offensive as any pissed adult.

John nods at the toddlers. 'Wonder how many of these cherubs will end up drunk in here one day,' he says.

'Shall we pick up coffee?' I suggest.

It's not even midnight and it feels like 3 am.

*

An hour later we treat an eighteen-year-old man who was driving home from a party with his girlfriend when he lost control of his car and smashed into the front of a house. He's covered in blood from several wounds to his face and is limping across the road with his girlfriend following behind.

The accident happened in a cul-de-sac, though we guess the impact occurred at nearly fifty kilometres per hour. The solid brick house is barely damaged, but the front of the car is crumpled to the dash and there are two neat halos in the windscreen made by human heads. Chances are the seatbelts were forgotten. Although the man insists he was driving, I see long hairs embedded in the windscreen on the driver's side and suspect it was, in fact, his girlfriend behind the wheel and that she was over the limit, so they decided to try to con us.

'Any drugs with your drink?' John asks the man when the cop has turned his back.

'Just the usual,' he replies with a smirk.

'What's the usual?'

'Coke, meth, ecstasy, you know . . .'

We call for a second ambulance to sort out the girl. Then we lay her boyfriend on our stretcher with a neck brace on and John climbs into the back with him. All the way to hospital the young man talks through a plot to stop his parents finding out about the crash.

'I'll tell them I put the car in the workshop. Okay, so I won't have a licence for a while – well, so what? Dad'll lend me his Audi for work and I'll drive it round the block and park it and secretly catch the bus. I mean, I can do that for months, right? Months! They'll never know. Genius idea of mine, isn't it? Tell me I'm a genius. Hey you, ambo, you're not going to call my parents are you? I'm eighteen, you know. You can't call them, legally. I know my rights.'

John says he won't call them as long as he lies still and leaves his neck brace on and tries a bit harder to keep quiet.

'In your condition, you really shouldn't be talking,' John advises him.

John loves that line, it's one of his favourites. Talking hardly ever made a patient worse. But it can certainly grate on a weary paramedic. And at this time of night John is less than tolerant of a cocky rich kid trying to squirm his way out of a situation demanding he grow up and take responsibility.

Back at the station, at 3 am, I make us both a cup of tea, but John is snoring on the lounge before it's finished brewing. He loves that lounge; for me it's not quite long enough. In the next room I take off my rescue boots and lie on the bed. Getting comfortable is usually all we have time for.

Five minutes later the phone rings and we're up again.

I shake John as I pass the lounge. He pushes me away.

'You go,' he croaks, hugging a little pillow to his chest.

While paramedic work gets easier with time, our fourteen-hour night shifts don't. Even if we're lucky enough to shut our eyes for a moment we know that soon we'll be wrenched from sleep again, thrown into a brawl, a cardiac arrest, a pedestrian hit by a car. These sudden shots of adrenalin, the impact of the ups and downs, take years off our lives. Or so it feels. By the morning we can look as bad as our patients. And what's in store at the end of this career? Strokes, heart attacks, ulcers, dementia? Shift work is worse for the health than smoking. No wonder so few paramedics stay in the city as long as John and I have. So why do we stick around? Is it the buzz, the excitement of the place, the craziness we're drawn to? Whatever the reason, it's killing us slowly.

John reluctantly plods down the stairs to the ambulance.

As I step on the accelerator he says, 'Going a bit hard, aren't you?' His eyes are closed and I know he wants me to cruise so he can sleep as we drive. Last week we got a call at 2 am, and when I got behind the wheel I heard the side door open and shut and there was John curled up on the stretcher. I drove to a drunk in the gutter, gave the guy a nudge and sent him on his way. John slept through it all.

It might be tempting, the idea of sleeping on the stretcher. But it's not for me. The blood and vomit and faeces I've seen it covered in makes it less than inviting.

'The controller reckons it's a traumatic cardiac arrest,' I say, hoping this'll wake John up.

'Bullshit,' he murmurs, eyes still closed.

'I'm serious.'

He sighs and blinks and reaches for gloves.

*

In a wealthy suburb, at the bottom of a narrow, winding road, we see the flash of police beacons by the harbour's edge. We arrive in the driveway of a mansion of gigantic proportions: five storeys of ultra-modern luxury, with glass balconies all round and an open garage containing several classic cars.

'Oh God,' John says. He's not reacting to the opulence of the house but to the scene lit by the beam of our headlights.

Ahead of us are two police officers doing CPR on a middle-aged woman. We get out and step over a syrupy trail of blood coming from her head. The policewoman doing chest compressions looks up at us, her ponytail flicking to and fro. She's far too breathless to say anything. I tell her to continue what she's doing and I snip the woman's clothes off with my shears. John opens the defibrillator pads and sticks them on the patient's chest: one just below the right shoulder, the other under her left armpit.

'Hold it for a sec,' he says, lifting a hand.

Everyone stops, and we gauge the rhythm.

'Asystole,' John announces.

A flatline. No surprises there. An occasional blip crosses the screen, the heart's dying throes, a stray electrical charge. But there's no pulse. The woman's dead.

'What happened?' asks John.

The police officers shrug. There's a great deal of blood and the woman's arms are flaccid, her legs at awkward angles. Like me, John's seen these kinds of injuries before. Both of us look up at the towering mansion above.

'She's gone from the top,' says John, shaking his head.

It's a suicide, most likely. But the police need to rule out an accident, even murder. Whatever the case, our work is done. The woman's pupils are fixed and dilated and they're staring right through us. Her injuries are, as we say, 'incompatible with life'.

'A quick way to go,' says John, packing the gear.

I disagree. It's too hard to know. She could've been agonising for ages on the edge. 'Could've been hours of torture up there before she went over,' I say.

As we sit in the ambulance writing up the paperwork, a cop comes over and asks John if he'll speak to the husband. John nods reluctantly. One paramedic will always have to impart the bad news, and tonight I'm the driver so it's John. I step out and follow him into the house.

The woman's husband, flanked by two constables, is waiting for us. John doesn't speak; his face says it all. The man crumples to the floor, crying like a child. John crouches down beside him, puts a comforting hand on his back. It's all he does: just a hand, resting there. A minute goes by before the man gets up again. John guides him to the street, past the body of his wife covered with a sheet, across the river of blood. I go to pull the sheet off in case he wants to say goodbye. But his face is wracked by such terrible grief I know he doesn't have the strength to see her now, not in the state she's in. John almost carries him to the police car. The man will go to the station and make a statement, ring some relatives, friends. Meanwhile, the forensics team will photograph his wife where she lies before the contractors take her off in their van. After that, if they think of it, the constables guarding the scene will hose her blood into the harbour.

'Glad it's us tonight,' says John when we're back in the ambulance. 'Others might've worked on her.'

'Dreamers,' I say.

'So glad you're not a hero,' he says, driving away.

Honesty is the least we can offer. I've always felt uncomfortable trying to revive the patients we know are too far gone, all for the sake of the loved ones. Do we 'go through the motions' to show we've done our best? It's a nice idea. But does it help? Is it ethical?

'People think we raise the dead,' John says. And I know he also wonders, as I do, if it's worth the emotional toll on us, the paramedics burdened by the expectation of miracles.

CHAPTER 4

Four days off can rocket past like an ambulance, so it's vital to make them last, to savour every moment. It takes a while to bounce back from the night shifts though, a day or two at least. Those days are for slow walks, reading in the park, going to the movies. Up until a month ago those days would've also been for a date with Kaspia at Fu Manchu, our favourite local diner.

But my days off don't rocket past at all. Time stretches endlessly before me and I'm unsure what to do with it. Kaspia told me our break would make us more creative and productive. She said she'd lost herself, and was living in my shadow. Time apart would enable me to write more, and she'd be able to focus on a show she was planning to put on in January. As a burlesque dancer, she usually performed for a company called Sugartime in a popular monthly vaudeville directed by

Russall S. Beattie. But she wanted to produce her own show, and after that explore her other creative talents.

So I agreed to the split, wanting to be supportive, and picturing myself writing a novel without disturbance in just a few months. I imagined evenings surrounded by laughing artists and poets, sipping cocktails on my balcony overlooking the city lights, jazz musicians jamming in my lounge room.

Instead I'm weighed down by a loneliness that makes me good for nothing. When I try to write, the words don't come. No one calls, and late at night I lie awake and listen to the sirens going up and down Oxford and Victoria to St Vinnies, reminding me that I'll soon be back at work again, and that maybe it's a good thing.

On day three I drag myself out of bed and drive my car to Bondi, this time not for work. Above a shoe shop there's a music school where I learn guitar. I ring the doorbell and my teacher, Paul, a bald man in his fifties, lets me in. He smiles and shakes my hand.

'Hey mate, come on up.'

Paul plays piano and a dozen other instruments. On guitar he's the best I've ever seen. There are videos of him on YouTube where his fingers move so fast they seem to disappear.

I first met Paul on a frigid morning at The Gap. He'd climbed the fence at the crack of dawn. For a while it was only him and me, and he told me about the tragic events that had led him to this point. He and his wife of ten years both suffered depression, but his wife's was more severe. It was so debilitating for her that all she ever talked about was suicide. She'd regularly send him messages while he was with his music students, threatening to kill herself. Paul would end his lessons early and hurry home to stop her. He was in a constant state of worry about finding her dead one day, a worry that compounded his own depression and suicidal thoughts.

One winter night Paul woke up and saw that his wife was gone. He got out of bed and found her hanging in the bathroom. She'd made herself all pretty, as if for a night on the town, wearing her favourite dress and lipstick, hair brushed back. Paul ran into the street, screaming hysterically. The police had to tackle him to the ground. He was in what is known as a 'grief psychosis' and needed sedating.

As if this wasn't tragic enough, Paul told me his adult children blamed him for their mother's death, suggesting he'd driven her to suicide with his own dark moods. It took him a long time to face the world again.

Months after I met Paul at The Gap I spoke to him on Bondi Beach. He was jogging on the soft sand in the middle of the day, when the sand is hot as coals. It wasn't the first time I'd seen him there but I decided to join him for a bit, running beside him for just a minute or so, to see how he was getting on. He remembered me and shook my hand, although he wouldn't stop; he had to keep going. 'It's my therapy,' he said as he ran. Then he asked me if I played an instrument. I told him I played piano but wanted to learn guitar. He offered to give me some lessons, the first one for free, his way of thanking me for my help.

'Where'd we get up to?' he asks, turning a pencil between finger and thumb. He scrawls a series of chords in my workbook. 'These are the ones from last time, right?'

I nod. I'm worried he'll be disappointed, as I haven't practised much this week. My chord changes are slow, but I manage to strum them out.

'Not bad,' he says. 'More work needed though.'

I'm suddenly conscious of becoming another burden in Paul's life, a student who never improves.

Befriending a patient is an ethical minefield, especially with the mentally unwell, and is strongly discouraged for a range of reasons that I appreciate. But the professional divide between the paramedic and the patient is not necessarily a positive, in my view. It's too easily mistaken for a divide between the strong and the weak, the sane and the mad. It's a hierarchy that perpetuates stigmas. Although I sometimes ask Paul if he's going okay, I never play the paramedic with him. When I'm in his studio it's all about the music. He might once have been my patient, but now I'm his student. We all have something to give one another.

The only other time I've kept in contact with a psychiatric patient is with a man I met at The Gap, three years ago. There was something sacred about that meeting, something I couldn't walk away from. His name was Stephen. He jumped from the highest point, confirmed by witnesses. We spotted him floating off the rocks, waving at us. We couldn't believe our eyes. It's true that it was high tide, a king tide in fact. Even so, it defied all rational explanation. Survivals are just so rare.

The water police picked him up ten minutes later and we met the launch at the Watsons Bay marina. Stephen was conscious but drowsy, and both his legs and pelvis were fractured. He was deathly pale, his blood pressure at rock bottom. He was losing blood internally but we got a line and started fluids, then splinted him as best we could for the urgent trip to hospital.

The next day we went to visit Stephen in the ward and gifted him a lottery ticket. It was John's idea, not mine. Stephen's parents were at his bedside and shook my hand. I couldn't help but ask him to confirm that he'd gone from the top. He nodded. I asked him what, if anything, he was thinking as he fell. A recent *New York Times* article on suicide jump survivors in the US had claimed that most changed their minds mid-flight. Stephen told me the drop was almost too quick for thought, but he did remember a flash of regret the moment he fell. Was it a change of mind, I asked? Stephen paused for a minute, then nodded. Yes, he said, it was. It was also a kind of awakening. This idea was consistent with a study in the seventies of those who'd survived a jump and spoke about having 'transcendence' and a 'spiritual rebirth'. Stephen's mother said she believed an angel broke her son's fall.

A week later a case of Tooheys Red was delivered to the ambulance station, a gift from Stephen's father. He must have known there was nothing better at the end of a long summer shift dealing with suicidal people than a cold beer on the verandah. It was a timely present as we'd just run out of beers donated by another patient, a man who'd assaulted us while drunk and woken up the following day feeling guilty about it. Kind of ironic, really, our compensation arriving in the form of the beverage that got the guy in trouble in the first place.

Six months later I called up Stephen's dad to see how his son was. I didn't have Stephen's number; if I did I would've called that instead. His father told me Stephen believed he was *selected* to live, and that his ambition was to find his true purpose. He was studying and working and seeing a girl. He was doing very well.

Occasionally, when I'm speaking to people on the edge, I mention one of these names. Paul, the musician, still alive, sharing his music with the world, including me. And Stephen, the one who jumped and changed his mind.

On the morning of my first day back at work I'm feeling agile, upbeat, ready for anything. Being in the ambulance is a million times better than moping around feeling sorry for myself for messing up my relationship with Kaspia. John, on the other hand, comes in late and doesn't look well. He plods up the stairs like a geriatric, every step an effort. He's badly hungover.

'Countersign the drugs and we're good to go,' I say.

After a double-shot latte we pick up an eighty-year-old woman with cellulitis from a mouldy ground-floor apartment. Her name's Nancy. As we carry her into Casualty she tells us she could've been a big-time singer.

'My father, he wanted to make me famous,' she says. 'But I kept having epileptic fits on stage and a mean girl stole my piano music.' To prove her talent, Nancy faces a packed emergency waiting room and sings 'My Funny Valentine'. She has a raw and croaky voice, but it's strangely beautiful in an unpolished way. When she's done, her audience of sick and injured people manages a meek applause.

She says to John, 'You know, the other night my father was in my dream and told me he was coming into the world again. So I went out and bought a box of disposable nappies and a little blue jumpsuit for a baby boy.'

'Well?' John asks her. 'Did your father show up?'

'No, he didn't. A terrible shame,' replies Nancy, downcast. 'I reckon the carpet turned him off. He always hated the carpet in our place. I can only blame myself. After all these years I never ripped it up.'

A drunk man calls for an encore from Nancy, but she's sombre now. We've taken the song right out of her. In youth it's easy to say we don't have regrets. The future is long, full of promise and dreams. We've got less to look back on, less to weigh up, more time left. But old age is marked by quiet, by slow days and weeks and years for reflecting on what life was, what it wasn't, what it might have been. Health problems are just one discomfort. Regret is painful too. And many regrets are worse than not becoming a famous singer. Old age has few upsides, especially if your partner has passed away before you. No wonder John talks of dying in his 'prime'. His worst nightmare is to be on his own in old age, to die with no one beside him. There aren't many health workers I know who aspire to longevity. If those who make toasts to long lives understood what this actually entailed, they'd keep their mouths shut.

John throws the ambulance into oncoming traffic. We hurtle down the wrong side of New South Head Road to upmarket Bellevue Hill. The eyes of approaching drivers widen in horror. An ambo with a death wish, some might be thinking. Normally he's cautious, always the one to slow *me* down. 'Going a bit hard, aren't you?' he'll say when I push it. But now it's John who's swerving around the banked-up cars at busy intersections in a way that makes me nauseous.

As we miss the mirror of a delivery truck by a whisker, John blurts out, 'Fucking Antonio!' and leans on the horn.

'You okay, mate?' I have to raise my voice to be heard above the siren.

'It's bullshit!'

'Has he left?'

'Two days ago. Walked out.'

Why hadn't he told me this earlier?

'I'm sorry,' I say. 'I gather you were drinking on your own then, last night?'

'I always drink on my own. Antonio doesn't like it.'

I remember John telling me about Antonio coming home from work and finding him sloshed on the lounge with the sun still up. He wasn't impressed. Our colleague Jerry, who's known John longer than I have, reckons his drinking got bad after one of his nephews died a year ago. It was a tragedy that cut John to the core. The son of his sister was only nineteen and just coming out as gay, trying to make sense of his feelings and place in the world. His Uncle John was pretty much his only confidant, someone who understood him and could help him grasp his sexuality and the daunting prospect of sharing it with his parents and friends. But then one day, while John and Antonio were on a holiday in Rio, the teenager stepped in front of a train. He was killed instantly. John was devastated, and he blamed himself for a while, as most people do in such cases. Blamed himself for not having been there, not paying attention when he was needed most.

John rarely brings up the topic of his nephew anymore. Not because he doesn't think about what happened; of course he does. But it's hard remaining composed and useful in a job like ours while focused on our personal grief. It's a compassion competition, and compassion for our patients and their relatives trumps compassion for ourselves. If it didn't, I guess we'd probably quit. If self-compassion came first, wouldn't it be sensible for us to stay at home and avoid getting tangled in the turmoil of strangers?

John pulls up at a red-brick house with a carefully tended hedge out front. It's the only 1930s house left in a street of newly built mansions. We take our gear through the open door and down a hallway. In the lounge room a group of relatives stand and look at us. Beside them is a truly horrendous sight: an elderly woman crushed by a wooden cupboard. She must have severed an arterial vessel because there's blood up the walls, right to the ceiling. We're no detectives but we speculate she tripped and fell on the carpet, grabbing at the open cupboard door and pulling the whole thing onto herself.

Despite the graphic nature of the scene and her violent death, the family is oddly composed. One of the woman's daughters-in-law even comments, 'She was so unwell, you know; it's probably for the best she's dead. Couldn't be more perfect, really.'

Couldn't be more perfect, really? This might be a reasonable thing to say about someone who'd peacefully slipped away in their sleep. But a grandma crushed by a cupboard?

John and I glance at one another, which is enough to see the other is equally appalled by the relative's attitude.

John doesn't hesitate to get bossy with the family. 'I think we all need to leave the room. It's a crime scene until proven otherwise. Thank you. The police are on their way.'

We wait for the cops in the air-conditioned ambulance and try to guess what the relatives are discussing in whispers out the front.

'Market value of the property,' says John.

'Without a doubt,' I reply.

We manage to get a second coffee before we're sent to 'a female held hostage' in a Bondi apartment. Kidnapping's not the kind of call we get that often, so it sparks our interest.

As we pull up at the address John's phone pings with a message from Antonio. John starts texting furiously. 'I'll wait here,' he says with agitation. 'You handle the kidnapping.'

I leave him be and get out and squeeze past a couple of cop cars then walk up the narrow staircase of the unit block.

Inside the apartment two constables are questioning a man in his thirties who's sitting on the ground. I look around at the apartment, which is filthy and dank. There's no furniture except for a dusty computer on the floor and piles of DVDs lying around. A fold-out plastic Christmas tree is on its side and most of the windows are boarded shut.

One of the constables approaches and says, 'Bloke here met a girl from Prague on a dating site. Convinced her to live in Australia. Paid for her flight, picked her up from the airport, brought her here. But he wouldn't let her go. She's been locked in that room there for a month.' The cop points to an adjacent bedroom. 'In the end she cut her wrists and he freaked out when he saw the blood and called for help. That's the lowdown, mate.'

In a corner of the bedroom I find the woman with lacerations and marks from being tied up. The wounds aren't deep, but I dress them anyway. She speaks no English, and all I can do is gently guide her down the stairs and into the ambulance. Through tinted windows we watch the cops escort her kidnapper to a cage truck for his own taste of captivity. He's pumped up, sweating, red in the face. There must have been a struggle after we left the room because gold tinsel from the guy's two-dollar Christmas tree is entangled in his handcuffs and trails along behind him, twinkling in the midday sun. The police push him into their wagon, and one of the constables picks up the end of the tinsel and tosses it in behind him. The constable slams the door shut and we hear him say, 'Merry fucking Christmas, dickhead!'

At St Vincent's I eat a falafel roll in the ambulance and think about the kidnapping. Every case of domestic violence I've encountered, every terrible story of romance gone wrong, makes me reflect on the relative harmony and stability of my relationship with Kaspia. Maybe we were fine all along, but simply didn't see it. The good times were many. How could we forget? We'd journeyed through Indian deserts by motorbike, across Bulgarian mountains by car, into Moroccan villages by bus. We'd seen the world together, danced together, laughed together. Our lives were entwined in an epic story deserving of a happy ending. So what happened? Did we take each other for granted? Did we get bored when our world adventures ended and we settled back in Sydney?

I want to call her and say hi, see how she's going. But then I notice John on his phone pacing around the ambulance bay, shaking his head and gesticulating, and I know he's talking to Antonio. This is quite likely the way my conversation with Kaspia would go if I broke our no-call agreement, and I decide it's not worth it.

When John finishes his call he gets back into the front passenger seat and I hand him a mini apple juice and hospital sandwich. He likes hospital sandwiches, which I can't stomach. Though he nods in thanks, he's too distracted to be hungry and puts my gift in the side door for later.

'I'm moving out,' he declares.

'What?'

'Antonio can stay in the house. I'm packing my things.'

'Really?'

'Well *you* moved out, didn't you? Now it's my turn.'

'Where will you go?'

John sighs. 'No idea. I might call Missionbeat.' He lets out a short laugh without smiling at the idea of being collected by the city's homeless van. But it's not so silly. We've both met doctors, lawyers and corporate types living rough. Any of us could end up on the street. A personal tragedy, a few bad decisions or one bad job is all it would take.

'My place is pretty small, a kind of studio, but the lounge is yours,' I offer.

'You kidding me? Two miserable fuckers in one joint? I don't think so. I need privacy.'

'You sure that's a good idea?' But he ignores my question, or he's too deep in thought to hear. A second later we're interrupted by a call to Victoria Street anyway.

No time to manage our own shit, no time for resolution.

Always another call, another call, another call . . .

*

On approaching the scene we see there's a man lying in the middle of the road outside the Holiday Inn. He's surrounded by the 'circle of death', a ring of curious bystanders, none of whom are actually assisting him. The man is spread-eagled and not breathing.

'Old-fashioned heroin OD,' says John, pulling back the man's eyelids to show me pinpoint pupils.

Once, in 2000 when I was posted to Paddington for a roster, there was so much heroin on the streets we'd often run out of Narcan, the opiate antidote. Some days we treated half a dozen people for heroin overdoses back to back, reviving them in back alleys scattered with used needles, in dingy share houses and brothels. One particular case back then rattled me so much I had to leave the job for a while. A sixteen-year-old Indigenous girl we'd treated for overdoses two nights in a row wound up dead three weeks later in a doorway. It was unclear if she'd overdosed again and not been found for some time, or if someone had killed her. Her death was a real wake-up call for the health and social services that had failed her.

When the Kings Cross medically supervised injecting centre opened in 2001, driven by the need for a practical and compassionate harm-reduction measure, heroin deaths plummeted. Ambulance calls to the area for overdoses dropped by eighty per cent. It couldn't have come at a more important time.

John draws up Narcan from the drug kit and injects the man's deltoid while I ventilate his lungs. As I'm doing this I suddenly sense a gust of cold air creep down my collar. I look up and see a lanky man with reptilian features staring at us. It's a hot summer's day but he's wearing a black velvet cloak, black gloves and hat. For some strange reason I convince myself the man is Death himself, come to pick up another soul. I'm mesmerised for a moment, but soon the spell is broken by a moan from our patient, who starts to wake up. The stranger in black gives a guttural snarl and takes a step forward. His voice is croaky and he lets out a sarcastic growl: 'Fucken heroes, saving junkies!' He spits on the ground in disgust. Then with a flourish of coat-tails he turns on his heels and walks down the road. We watch as our patient, now conscious, follows behind.

John says the man was just a local weirdo; he's seen him before. He tells me I've got an active imagination. And he reckons he isn't scared of death, but I don't believe him. A while ago he told me that all of his basketball team in the eighties died of complications from AIDS, except him, and that he always expected he'd be next. He might've been scared of death back then, he admits. He can't believe he survived. He still wonders if he's invincible, or 'unkillable', as some of us describe a patient whose survival, or repeated survival, defies explanation.

'Would you ever do heroin?' I ask John.

'Of course I'd do it! Just don't like the idea of *injecting* it.'

'You know you can smoke it.'

'We *all* know that. Stop tempting me.'

'So you'd take heroin knowing you'd become a slave to it?'

'Right now I don't give a shit. Make me a slave.'

'It'll ruin your life.'

'What life?'

For a few minutes John sits quietly in thought. Then he breaks the silence with his own question for me.

'Would you consider a hot-shot of heroin if you wanted to kill yourself?'

I nod. 'Probably.'

'Right, so don't get on your high horse.'

I apologise.

'Problem is,' says John, 'if you wanted to end your life that way, you'd have to come down to Kings Cross here and loiter around like a junkie trying to score off some dodgy scumbag.'

'You'd lose momentum.'

'Exactly. You'd loiter around and get jack of it and go home, and feel twice as suicidal for fucking up your own suicide.'

Losing momentum might apply to impulsive suicides. But some people plan their deaths as carefully as others plan weddings.

'Let's change the subject,' says John.

'Good. Come stay at my place,' I say.

'No chance,' he says. 'I've got shit to sort out.'

*

Just off Riley Street, a cleaning lady has found a dead man. He's maybe forty years old, tubby, with a moon face. He looks Italian, maybe Greek. He's lying sideways on a cream shag-pile carpet and is wearing giant headphones. The room is cluttered with oil paintings, sculptures, piles of books, sheet music and cans of food. It's a tableau of isolation.

'Death by loneliness . . . what d'you reckon?' I say to John.

As soon as I've said it I know I shouldn't have. Not when he's about to move out on his own. But he doesn't react. He just stands and stares at the body for half a minute before going off to comfort the cleaning lady, who's crying in the hall. Watching John put his arm around her makes me think of the New York paramedic from Martin Scorsese's film *Bringing Out the Dead* who described himself as a 'grief mop'. John's the grief mop today, and God knows he isn't in any condition for it.

The dead man's skin is mottled, and the intense pungency in the room suggests he might've been dead for days. When I go to put a sheet over his body I can hear a symphony playing at full volume through the headphones still firmly on his head. The dial on the stereo is tuned in to Classic FM. What exactly was he listening to as he breathed his last, I wonder? What orchestral piece played while his heart petered out? How lucky this man would've been if his death had been accompanied by a gentle, angelic lullaby.

★

We park on the side of Stanley Street near the famed Italian restaurant Bill & Toni's so I can write up the case sheet. John spies one of his friends leaning against a four-wheel drive. The man has a big, bushy beard and hairy forearms. It's the fuzzy look so many gay men are going for these days. When John returns to the ambulance I'm pleased to see him looking brighter.

'That's Terry. He was just in a gay bar up the road, says he was hit on by a bloke in a Ned Kelly helmet. I told him only ugly gays wear helmets.'

I laugh. 'I'll remember that.' I tell him about my own family's history with the Kelly gang in Victoria, and he smiles. I wonder if Ned Kelly ever imagined he'd become an Australian gay icon a hundred and fifty years later.

On the way back to the station we drive along Oxford Street and I see one of Kaspia's friends, Gypsy Wood, a burlesque dancer from Sugartime, walking up the road. Her mother named her after Gypsy Rose Lee, the American striptease artist of the forties, and she does a great routine as the absinthe fairy with green feather fans. John knows Gypsy too. They met last week, when we stopped by a pool party at the Bondi share house where she lives with dancers from the Australian Ballet.

As we pass Gypsy, I whoop the siren at her. She spins around and lifts up her skirt to flash her underwear. Kaspia would've done the same, I know that. How quickly I've forgotten her sense of fun, especially in public. She spontaneously dances and sings in the street at the top of her voice and can imitate anyone, her impressions always spot on. Her laughter is raucous.

John blows Gypsy a kiss, and she waves as we pass.

After a couple more cases we're dispatched to Ken's of Kensington, a sauna for gay men south of the city. Behind the chocolate-brown entrance is a world unknown to most passers-by. It's a dim and foggy maze of partitioned cubicles, with men young and old wearing little red towels and pairing off for sex. While waiting for a partner many men loiter about completely naked, openly flaunting Viagra-charged erections.

John has been here before, sent on a job, he insists, never for pleasure. While drugs of abuse are banned at these venues, we're often called to accidental overdoses on gamma hydroxybutyrate, or GHB, which most of us refer to simply as 'G'. This liquid intoxicant popular among gay men enhances sensuality, but doses are difficult to measure and the drug can easily put people in a coma.

The manager who meets us at the door is a hyperactive German with a military buzz cut who looks like a classic Tom of Finland sketch. He leads us to the patient, cursing all the way.

'Olvays I tell zem, no drucks! No drucks in here! If zey take ze drucks, I kick zem out. Zis guy, I am bannink him from Ken's. I'll make sure of zis. Dirty drucks is *not* vot Ken vonts.'

The body of our patient is slippery with fluids I dare not contemplate. When I lift his arm for a blood-pressure check it slides right out of my grip. John seems more adept at handling the man and dries him off with the little towel that was, until moments ago, tied around his waist like a loincloth. None of the other punters seem the least bit inclined to cease their activities. As one of their own lies critically ill, the grunting and groaning goes on. We work to this soundtrack while men keep arriving and departing around us. Hungry eyes stare down and I feel we're a sideshow, another live act in this fantasy-land. On a screen in the corner there's a film being played: two thrusting chefs, both covered in pasta. There's so much going on around me that it takes more than a minute to see the floor we are on is made of perspex and fully transparent, allowing a view to the level below where musclebound men cavort in a pool.

When I get home I take a shower and wash off the smell of the sauna. I realise I'm too tired to cook, so I just make some toast and hunt for a beer. There's none in the fridge, and I'm in no mood to go out again. I pour myself a whisky and put on a record. It's one Kaspia left behind, or rather one I *kept* when she left me: Björk's *Vespertine*. It was on high rotation in 2001, when we first fell in love. Now I'm next to the turntable and play 'Hidden Place', the song she loves most, and I play it again and again, until it's not Björk anymore but Kaspia singing.

CHAPTER 5

John doesn't turn up for his shift the next day. Instead when I walk into the station I find Jerry in a headstand position, a yoga asana, wearing nothing but jocks. I tiptoe around him, not daring to disturb his deep nasal breathing, his intense meditation. He was once a self-described 'pothead' before he turned into a yogi. Now he does yoga before every shift, sometimes even during. The headstand is Jerry's favourite pose. He says it's good for stress and depression, being upside down.

I make my tea as quietly as I can. When Jerry's done and his feet are back on earth, he says, 'I'm John for the day, in case you didn't notice.'

'John would never stand on his head,' I reply.

'Half his problem,' says Jerry, rolling up his mat.

'Did he call in sick?'

'A late swap. He's run out of sickies, taken too many. I spoke to him round midnight. He was packing the car. Totally pissed, of course. He's moving into one of Mick's units.'

Mick, a paramedic from Randwick, owns a few properties in the area. He got into real estate a decade ago, before the prices shot up. One of his flats in Bondi Junction is between tenants, and he offered it to John on a temporary basis.

'How did he sound?'

'Who? John?'

I nod.

'Like shit.'

We're a tight-knit team at Bondi, but Jerry's closer to John than I am. They occasionally swim down at Clovelly together, do laps of the inlet where people go snorkelling.

Jerry's a man of contrasts. He's a larrikin who hates the rulebook, but his shirts are always pressed. He adores his wife and children, but flirts with other women, even his elderly patients. He's committed to his yoga, but loves the football too. He'll read books on philosophy, then study the racing form guide. He knows how to stir and crack people up as well as John does.

We head out for coffee. Our favourite barista Dan is on shift at Gertrude & Alice, a bookshop café.

'What a fabulous day!' announces Jerry. 'Who'd call an ambulance on a day like this? Tell me, would you get out of bed on such a glorious morning and look out the window and think, *Ya know what? I'd like to spend my day in hospital while the doctors decide what to do with me.*'

That's Jerry all over. He puts a smile on your dial and keeps it there. If only John was rostered with him. Jerry's just the man he needs right now.

Before we can order coffee we're diverted to a guy sitting on a park bench, still drunk from the night before. Weekend mornings often start this way, with comedowns and hangovers.

The paralytic man snores on the stretcher beside me as we drive him to hospital, cruising past the beach to check out the surf. I gaze through the tinted windows, watching the swaying palms go by. At the next set of lights I see a woman in a yellow bikini waiting to cross.

Jerry calls out to me from the driver's seat, 'Who's that Latino Hollywood actress? You know the one. With the big bum?'

I can't think.

'The girl at the lights there looks just like her, I swear it's probably her. Jennifer someone . . .'

The patient stirs beside me for the first time. With eyes still closed he croaks, 'Lopezzzzz,' then drops back unconscious, or so he'd have us believe.

'That's it! Lopez!' Jerry snaps his fingers. 'Don't you reckon the girl at the lights looks like Jennifer Lopez?'

'A little bit,' I say.

Normally Jerry tries getting out of working Saturdays because he hates missing the horseraces. But he's here for John, filling in for his mate who's doing it tough.

It's a big race day, too. Jerry asks me to drop him off at the TAB when it opens so he can lay a few bets. A TAB is not a 'licensed establishment', he insists when I question him about wearing his uniform into a gambling joint. Like John, he doesn't care for spoilsports.

Race days with Jerry are painful. As if driving with a siren wailing in one ear and race commentary in the other isn't distracting enough, Jerry cheers the horses and punches the air beside me as we go.

'Bastard! I had fifty on that Cream Cake,' he curses as I mount another median strip and narrowly miss a bus. The passengers are probably thinking he's cursing the traffic.

Thankfully, later in the morning, Jerry wins a bet on a horse called Course Ya Can, which settles him down.

'Knew I'd get lucky with that one,' he says.

'How's that?'

'You know, when patients ask me, "Can I come to hospital?" I always say, "Course ya can!" and if they say, "Can I have some morphine?" I say, "Course ya can!" too. It's the kind of man I am. That's why I picked the horse. Terrific name, isn't it? Sometimes a name just clicks, you know? I'll pick a horse for that reason.'

After waiting fifteen minutes outside another TAB, I say, 'What about blackjack? Will you ask me to stop at the casino next?'

'Casino? We need to wait for a *call* to the casino first,' says Jerry. 'It's out of our catchment. Discretion is everything.'

'Discretion? Like parking an ambulance outside a TAB?'

'Fair cop, but casinos are different. What ya gunna do? Go up the escalators, push through the poker lanes, wait till the Chinese are only four deep at the table? No way. Ya can't do blackjack on the job. Too risky. We're an emergency service.'

'Least you might win something at blackjack. How much have you made today? Three dollars?'

Jerry's annoyed I've mocked his small win, so he goes and puts two hundred on a horse called Happy Choo-Choo. It's racing at 2 pm, but at 1.57 pm we get a call to a 'female collapsed'. Jerry knows he'll miss the race and he curses.

On a kitchen floor surrounded by crumbs lies Marjory, eighty years old. She fainted while taking a tray of Anzac biscuits out of the oven. She's got no idea an important horserace is happening.

'My cookies . . .' she murmurs as she comes to.

Marjory's daughter scolds her mother with a finger raised. 'Just let the nice men look you over, Mum. Forget about the cookies!'

But I find myself assessing Marjory alone. Jerry hovers by the patient's daughter and I overhear him saying, 'You know I'm very much a betting man and, ah, I happen to have some money on a horse today . . .'

'You do?' she replies. 'That's nice.'

'Yes, yes, I know. It's called Happy Choo-Choo, the horse. A handsome horse. A strong horse, strong and fast. In fact, it's running any second now.'

'It is?'

'Yes, it is. Any second. You wouldn't mind if I, ah, turned on this here television to see if Happy Choo-Choo wins the race?'

How readily and happily Marjory's daughter obliges him. Moreover, after switching on the TV set she makes a cup of tea for Jerry and brings it to him, along with a biscuit on a little blue plate. Meanwhile I'm taking Marjory's blood pressure, blood sugar, temperature and ECG. I try getting a history but my voice is drowned out by the shrill racing commentary overlaid by Jerry's emphatic cries of, 'Yes, Happy Choo-Choo! Go, Happy Choo-Choo, come on Happy Choo-Choo, go, damn it, Happy Choo-Choo! Go, you bloody beauty! Yes, yes, YES!'

And just as Marjory regains her colour, Jerry wins eight hundred dollars.

★

In the early afternoon there's a call about a cardiac arrest a block from the station. The patient's name is Harry, and he's seventy-five years old. His distraught wife recounts his final words before he fell unconscious: 'Damn this stupid cough!'

Harry has been down too long. We try reviving him but he doesn't respond. I'm hardly surprised. We rip a man's shirt off, jump on his chest, snap off some ribs, stick tubes down his throat, and for what in the end? All this action to have him stay dead, as most of them do. The whole song and dance, when survival's out of reach, insults a dignified life.

I tell Harry's wife that her husband has died and she covers her face with her hands and cries. She speaks to him through tears: 'Oh Harry, don't go, please . . . You were here just now. You said you'd give up drinking and smoking, said you'd look after us . . .'

I crouch down beside her, my arm round her shoulder, and look down at the expressionless face of her husband. Jerry goes to get her phone book so she can make some calls, let their adult children know their father is gone.

The man's last words repeat in my head.

Damn this stupid cough.

Last words are not important, not like they are in movies. I've never heard dark secrets or clues revealed. If anything, last words are banal. Even so, some of them I can't forget.

'I'm telling you it's undercooked, my dear.'

'Just pass the remote.'

'Anyone seen my pills?'

'Gotta go to the toilet.'

'Shut up, will you?'

'Stop annoying me.'

Sudden death rarely allows for lines like, 'I've always loved you, darling,' or 'The hour has come,' or 'Seize the day and believe in yourself, my son.'

It's a pity, really. If we lived a less profane existence, if we spoke more wisely always, our last words might count. Every other important life event, like our weddings and birthdays, is scripted. But death is most often a surprise. I don't so much fear death as fear it will be ordinary, or that I'll utter something stupid just before I'm taken.

Jerry buys me a coffee and we give John a call to check in. It goes to voicemail. We've taken only a sip of coffee when Control decides to send us to an asthma attack in Bondi.

'Went to a nasty asthma case with John the other day,' I say. 'She bloody died.'

Jerry leans across and flicks the siren on.

'Better make some noise then,' he says.

We fly past busy cafés, making such a racket that people put their fingers in their ears.

'Look at them,' Jerry scoffs, shaking his head. 'We sit here with the siren blaring day and night and these soft Bondi hipsters can't stand a few seconds.'

I take a wrong turn down a narrow one-way street and throw on the brakes. I try to reverse but three cars have lined up behind me.

'Hope the patient's not too crook,' says Jerry, unhelpfully.

On cue, our data terminal updates. Our patient is no longer breathing. A friend has started mouth-to-mouth.

'For fuck's sake, man. I thought you knew this street?' Jerry says. He opens his door and hops out. He walks back to direct the traffic behind us while I curse and begin reversing the ambulance with the siren still on.

Once we're out of the one-way trap it's only half a minute to the scene. Heaped with our gear, we plunge down the stairs of a unit block. On the concrete porch outside number two, a young man is lying on the ground surrounded by his friends. A pale girl with long hair is giving him the mouth-to-mouth. She looks up between each breath, her eyes pleading with us for help.

'You've done well,' I tell the girl. 'Stop there and let's see how he is.'

She backs away, wiping her mouth. 'His name's Billy. He didn't have his Ventolin. He said he was having an asthma attack; we didn't know what to do.'

But Billy is breathing just fine. His lungs are inflating with ease and there's no audible wheeze, not even a hint. Jerry gently runs a finger over the lashes of Billy's closed eyes. The lashes flutter in response, a sure sign he's not unconscious.

Jerry shakes his head. He hates people bunging it on, and is clearly pissed off. But we have to be sensitive in how we resolve it. I lean down beside our patient and speak in a whisper so no one will hear.

'Now listen, Billy. We know you're a faker; I've seen a whole lot. We're pretty hard to fool. You have your reasons and we don't want to embarrass you. So what I'll do is put oxygen on your face and you can wake up, okay?'

Billy gives me a subtle nod and I crank on the cylinder and let him have a minute of oxygen.

'He'll pull through,' I announce to the group. 'Any second now he'll come round.'

Billy begins to moan. He stirs gradually, like all fakers do, as if emerging from under a spell. He rubs his eyes and looks around with comic-book confusion. 'W–w– . . . what happened? Where am I?' he asks. 'What're you all doing here?'

Together, Jerry and I escort Billy to his bedroom and close the door behind us.

'What's with the stunt?' I ask him.

'Sorry, I didn't think they'd actually call you.'

'You *did* tell them you were having an asthma attack.'

'It wasn't about that.'

'What then?'

'The girl.'

'The girl?'

'Christie. I've liked Christie for years and she won't go out with me. I can't stop thinking about her. Do you know what that feels like? To love someone and not be loved back? Anyway, she did a first-aid certificate a couple of weeks ago and, well, I got to thinking . . .'

'You wanted to be her patient? You wanted her to give you mouth-to-mouth?'

He nods. 'Kiss of life, yeah. But not just that. I wanted to see if she cared enough to, you know, save me from dying . . .'

Jerry sighs. I'm surprised he's so unimpressed. Faking an asthma attack to get kissed by a girl is something I could imagine Jerry doing as a teenager.

Billy looks ashamed. 'I really didn't think they'd call you. I was enjoying it, and before I knew it you were there and I was in too deep. You were so quick! I'm sorry. Please don't tell her I faked it, please . . .'

Some paramedics might contact the police at this point. But I like his sense of romance, his cheekiness. There's not enough of it about these days. I too have pulled some pranks for love in my time. Once, at Heathrow Airport, I turned up in a gorilla suit to surprise Kaspia at Arrivals.

As we walk out the door I glance back at Billy, who is sitting on the edge of his bed, a victim of unrequited love, tenderly licking his lips with a smile at the edge of his mouth.

*

It's mid-afternoon when a man goes under a train at Bondi Junction. Our control needs two crews for the case. My stomach is turning and I hope we're not the ones picked, but since we're the second-closest ambulance we're given the job. The only relief is that it's Jerry and me going, and not John. The similarity to his nephew's death could have been enough to tip him right over.

I don't do ambulance work for the gore, I never have. Even the thought of major trauma makes me sick. I still remember my first 'train job' on the North Shore Line. My palms were all sweaty, my heart beating hard. The man's headless body lay on the tracks: just a torso and a leg. I found a pair of shoes and his mobile phone ten metres from his body. An audio message blinked on the screen, a suicide statement we played then and there. In the message he listed the people he loved and he sobbed through each name. He apologised for dying in the way that he had.

We put a sheet on his body and searched for his head. We looked along the tracks, poked around in the shrubs nearby.

Plenty of people hit by trains will be thrown, their bodies intact. But if they go underneath, their injuries are horrendous and few will survive. Only those completely immersed in their own sadness and pain could forget about the emergency workers who will clean up their bodies.

We arrive at the station and go down the escalators to the underground platforms. An ambulance crew is already there and Mia from Paddington gives us a wave.

According to witnesses, an elderly man in a suit and bow tie has calmly walked forward into the path of a train.

'Where's your partner?' Jerry asks Mia.

'Crawling down there,' she says, pointing under the train.

'Is the guy still alive?'

She shrugs then calls out, 'Mandy! Hey, Mandy! Is he dead or alive?'

'Dead!' comes the reply.

A moment later we hear Mandy again, sounding distressed.

'Oh my God! How disgusting!'

We all crouch and lean down, the police officers too, and imagine the worst.

'What is it?' calls Mia. 'You good?'

I'm glad it's just us who hear Mandy's reply.

'Chewing gum, damn it. Stuck to my pants!'

Everyone lets out a sigh of relief.

One suicide a day is plenty for me, but we don't get a choice to leave it at that. At six in the evening we're sent to The Gap for a girl on the edge. Suicides peak in the lead-up to Christmas; it's the same every year. But it's never this bad, and Jerry agrees.

We're late to the scene and glad the police have beaten us there. Down from the lighthouse the police rescue squad are rigging up ropes to their truck. There's nothing much else to tie off on up here. Plan A is to talk the girl down from her perch. Plan B is to grab her if she tries to go over.

Jerry checks the glovebox then slams it shut, annoyed.

'No Nobby's Nuts? You and John eat them all?'

I shrug. 'We've been here a lot.'

'Would be nice to buy more, don't you think?' Jerry says. 'It's part of restocking the car. Oxygen, cannulas, bandages, nuts.'

I remember a thing I've been meaning to ask him.

'You ever boiled frankfurters?'

'Frankfurters? Sure.'

'I boiled them last night and the jackets slipped off. I couldn't believe it.'

Jerry cranks his seat back, thinks for a second.

'Did you toss them right in?'

'Sure I did. Three at once.'

He's shaking his head, looking dismayed.

'What were you doing? Didn't you think to experiment first, to start with just one?'

'When the jackets came off I turned the heat down, but they'd already died.'

Jerry closes his eyes, summoning patience.

'You've got to start with your frankfurters immersed in the cold water, then increase the heat nice and slow. Understood?'

I nod.

A high-flying seagull gets my attention. I see it glide past the girl on the cliff and she watches it too, follows its course. It briefly hovers and turns to glance at the drama on the clifftop, then carries on its way.

'You could also get a stick and put it in the end of the frankfurter,' says Jerry, 'then roll it in beer batter and deep-fry it. Dagwood dog's what they call it. My brother and I, we had a tradition. Dagwood dogs on Golden Slipper Day. They don't sound that healthy, but they're bloody delicious.'

We see the girl climbing back over the fence and the police rescue guys leading her to us. We get out and meet her. I tell her she's done the right thing, choosing life. It's kind of presumptuous, but I mean it sincerely, and in any case it's what I'm paid to say. She asks for a tissue, so I hand her a few. But as we turn onto Old South Head Road her tears have turned to laughter as Jerry recounts my frankfurter story, and wonders aloud how a man like me can mess up a meal a child could prepare.

CHAPTER 6

If I were John I'd be taking nights off, not days. But he comes in for his graveyard shift, and not just any graveyard shift: it's a Friday night. He's a sucker for punishment, that's for sure. But I'm glad to see him.

'Sorry I didn't return your call,' he says.

'No worries. How's the new place?'

He grunts. 'Full of grandmas and stickybeaks. And the kitchen's a shoebox.'

Before John's breakup with Antonio, they often used to cook together in the spacious kitchen of their terrace, as Kaspia and I did in Bronte. It was one of their favourite pastimes.

'What's happening with Antonio?'

'Nothing's changed. Apart from moving out.'

'Let's have some fun tonight,' I say, trying to cheer him up. But the night starts badly.

We're sent to Little Bay, near the southern tip of the eastern suburbs, for a violent domestic. We don't go this far south ordinarily, but the local station is short a few cars. Sick leave on Friday nights is always hard to cover.

On the front porch of a cottage, a single orange globe is flickering with moths. The patient has seen us, and before we can knock she opens the door. She looks highly anxious when we enter the hall and fumbles to lock up behind us.

Shelly's her name, and her eyes dart around in fear. Her left cheekbone is bruised and her whole face is swollen. She winces as she limps; her left leg is injured. Tears flood her cheeks.

'He went totally mad,' Shelly cries. 'He just snapped then he hit me again and again.'

John helps Shelly sit on a chair in the hall. He's always so gentle, so tender with patients. How well he comforts others while he himself is so broken-hearted. Seeing his hand on Shelly's shoulder makes me wish there was someone to give him the same care.

John unzips the first-aid kit and pulls out a splint and bandages. With her good hand Shelly wipes strands of hair from her face. She looks at me and says, 'I did a bad thing.'

'What's that?'

'I locked him out of the house.'

We hear an ear-piercing bang and the splintering of wood. It's coming from a room off the hall. Seconds later there's the shattering of glass, a broken windowpane.

I take a step back, away from the sound.

John's roller bandage unravels to the floor.

'Fucking thing,' he says.

Shelly stops crying. Her expression is one of horror. She begins to whimper, her body shivering in fear.

'He's outside! He took his cricket bat, he's coming back, he wants to kill me, he *will* kill me, I know he will, he'll do it for real. He doesn't care. He'll kill the both of you as well, he's got it in him, I'm telling you! He'll do it!'

I slide my hand to the portable radio on my belt and push the duress button. Then, just to be sure I radio in a coded mayday: '402, Zero 1, Code 1!'

Another crashing sound comes, this time from the sunroom, then a loud voice growling and cursing outside.

'Gunna get you, bitch. You wait!'

Shelly grips my arm and her fingernails dig in. At the same time a shadow appears through the glass of the front door. A cricket bat shatters a small pane, spraying fragments onto the welcome mat.

The man takes another swing. We stand our ground.

Do I imagine we can take this guy on, me and John? I pick up a vase from a coffee table, thinking I might throw it. John looks sideways at me and raises an eyebrow. I put the vase back. John's strangely serene as the door is demolished in front of us by Shelly's angry husband. The man leans through the gap he's made with his bat and reaches around to open the door from the inside.

Then he steps into the house.

He's a hideous thug of a human. His face is puffed and crimson. Droplets of blood from shards of glass dot his arms and fall onto the floor. John edges Shelly behind himself to protect her. I imagine all variety of unpleasant ways the scene will play out. The man looks at our uniforms, our defiant stares. Neither John nor I makes any effort to speak to him, allowing our body language to communicate. Getting to Shelly will mean getting past us. Not that two clean-cut boys from Bondi station could offer much resistance beyond a few hopeless slaps. If Jerry was here he'd say, 'Go easy, mate. We're lovers, not fighters!' But John and I are lost for words.

A bead of sweat crawls down my back. I take a deep breath. The man's eyes flick left and right as he decides where to strike. The ticking of a kitchen clock amplifies the tension.

A moment later comes the sweetest sound: sirens, first one, then two, then three, all rapidly approaching. The man cocks his head like an animal hearing a hunter's footfall. He glares at us for a little longer then drops the cricket bat and lumbers down the front steps and into the dark.

As we take Shelly to hospital I suggest to John that we let our ambulance inspector know what's happened.

'You need counselling or something?' he asks.

'Maybe I will, later on. Maybe you too.'

'I don't need counselling. This is what we do.'

I'm surprised at John's suck-it-up attitude.

'Have you never seen a counsellor with Antonio?'

'You kidding? Honestly, I couldn't be fucked. Sitting there telling some stranger about our situation for an hour. Fifty sessions and thousands of dollars later and they might understand a fraction of the shit. Even then, what are they going to say? That we're just not meant for each other? Great. Money well spent, eh.'

'Might turn out differently . . .'

'Might not.'

'Glass half-empty?'

'Completely.'

John ends the conversation by slamming his case folder shut and turning up the stereo. I realise I'm in no position to lecture him about couples counselling. A year ago Kaspia and I saw a psychologist in a small, stuffy room, a weird old woman who wouldn't have looked out of place with a crystal ball in front of her. She was the one who told us that all couples' arguments were intimate, selling the idea of conflict as a positive. She had a few valuable insights, but we didn't go back. We gave up looking after that. Life's busy and counsellors cost money, and we weren't in the mood for shopping around. Although now I wish we had.

Earlier in the night I prayed for rain. A decent downpour douses violence, washes troublemakers off the streets. John says that even *he* would pray again if God answered such requests.

But there's no rain, no cool change. Only the heat rising. And booze, lots of it.

We're diverted to the city on what's called 'area cover'. All the other ambulances are occupied. We're the only resource left. Whatever happens now, it's ours.

Darlinghurst Road is thick with revellers. A young man from Double Bay has tripped on a Kings Cross gutter, spraining his ankle. Most drunks wouldn't consider falling over to be unusual. Alcohol does that to people, everyone knows. But some men with trivial injuries will make a show of it. As we load our patient into the ambulance he proudly waves to the rest of the man-pack he's been crawling the strip with. Then he takes out his mobile phone, looks through his contacts and picks a friend to call, informing them of his crisis.

'Shady? Is Shady there? Tell Shady I've been in a really bad accident. Oh, he's there? Okay, put him on. Shady, is that you? Shady, yeah, you'd better sit down, mate. Just sit down, okay, find a place to sit down, trust me. I have to tell you something and you might wanna sit down to hear it.'

The guy isn't joking.

John leans into the front of the ambulance and says, 'You think his ankle might be front-page news tomorrow?'

'Up there with the war in Iraq,' I reply.

When the guy gets off his phone John offers him pain relief.

'Oh, God yeah! Dude, the pain is, like, *so* bad, like, I really can't take it. I mean, I don't want to be a hero anymore, know what I mean?'

In my rear-vision mirror I see John looking earnest. 'You're right,' he says. 'Even heroes need a break. Let me give you some morphine.'

'Morphine?' He seems surprised.

'You *did* say your pain was, like, *so* bad, right?'

Little does the guy know that John is probably giving him pain relief in the hope it'll quieten him down. It's what I've heard some doctors call a 'shut up' dose.

We treat a performer at the casino after that, a fire-breather called 'Jaguar', whose hair has caught alight. Then a short time later we go to a man hit by a taxi near The Pleasure Chest, an adult store in the Cross. He's unconscious on the road.

I can see John's tired and it's only 11 pm. While I manage the patient's airway, John takes out his trauma shears and cuts along the seams of the guy's leather pants and jacket for better examination. Cutting along seams is no obligation, just a courtesy so motorcyclists and leather-bound men can get their garments sewn up again.

But when the man wakes in Emergency a few hours later, he turns out to be highly abusive, cursing and spitting at the nurses.

'And there I was, saving his jacket,' says John with regret.

The senior nurse overhears him. 'Don't worry, John darling,' he says. 'The guy was such a fuckwit we shredded his leathers in the pan room.'

John laughs, out loud. It's the first time I've seen his face light up in weeks.

I hang around the triage room as John completes his paperwork. I see an altercation developing between two of the casualties waiting to be seen.

'Mate,' says one to the other, 'you got blood on your head.'

'Yeah, well, guess what? *You* got blood on *your* head.'

'Are you fuckin' with me?'

'No, I'm not fuckin' with you, idiot. What I said was *you* got blood on *your* head!'

'For fuck's sake! I was just telling *you* that *you* got blood on *your* head and now you're fuckin' with me like some parrot.'

'Parrot? You calling me a parrot? Ah, just shut the fuck up.'

'Yeah?'

'Yeah.'

It's about to get physical. When I see security approaching I let myself out. There's always entertainment in the triage area. The hospital ought to sell tickets for seats on Friday and Saturday nights, perhaps to raise funds for much-needed equipment. Few live shows I've seen come close to the hijinks of Accident & Emergency. Only last week a girl off her chops on ecstasy amused us by making rounds of the department hugging and kissing every other patient, telling each one how beautiful they were and how much she loved them. For many, the care and attention she delivered was all they really needed. Even John got in line for some love. The girl hugged him for a good minute, as if she could tell he needed it most.

At midnight we bring in a sweet old woman in velvet slippers and floral nightgown who smells like lavender and stale urine. We suspect she has a UTI. We don't have a choice but to put her next to an agitated man affected by amphetamines and covered in sores.

John startles the triage nurse with his deadpan handover.

'This is Phyllis, seventy-eight years old, picked up from a rave dance party after taking speed and acid.'

The nurse knows John too well. She giggles and playfully slaps his arm. My partner's sense of humour and his friendship with staff once again win us a bed for our patient. As we hand Phyllis over I feel the night is about to ramp up. Another crew arrives doing CPR on a man while a guy in the waiting room punches the triage window, yelling, 'Do I need to be shot to get a doctor?'

We slip out the doors and back into the ambulance.

Kings Cross is getting busy and our controller wants us down there. Revellers have spilt onto the road, and we creep along carefully. By this time of night no one seems to care about the traffic anymore. Alcohol has claimed the streets. Distracted by strippers in dressing-gowns outside Showgirls, I almost run over an old man with a walking stick who's crossing in front of us.

'Look at this guy,' I say to John. 'He's at least eighty, cruising the strip at 1 am.'

'Viagra,' says John.

Further down the road comes another unlikely spectacle: a family as wholesome as the Brady Brunch going into a strip club. There's a neatly groomed dad, well-dressed mum, teenage daughter and two teenage sons, all sauntering casually into the Pink Pussycat as if it were McDonald's.

'Tell me that's not strange,' I say.

'Not at all,' replies John. 'It's little Jimmy's eighteenth, and this is what he's been wishing for, or maybe his dad thinks he *needs* to see a strip show, you know, to be a man.'

But what about the mother and sister? The scene reminds

me of a family in Maroubra charged last week with illegal graffiti. Both parents and their kids were caught by police with spray cans and marker pens tagging walls at 3 am.

As we turn into Macleay Street we see a policewoman we know dragging a rough-looking man into a cage truck. I wind down the window and call out to her, 'What's going on?'

'Motherfucker spat in my eye!' she barks.

We keep driving and a trans woman dressed like Amy Winehouse, in a tight zebra-print pencil skirt and silver stilettos, gives us a wave. John waves back. Then I swing into a darkened laneway for a loop of the block but have to slam on the brake to avoid hitting two big men, one giving the other vigorous oral sex.

'Laneways are a thing, you know,' says John, matter-of-factly.

The men ignore the beam of our headlights and carry on their antics without the slightest effort to let our ambulance pass. I've no interest in watching them, waiting for them to finish, so I back out of the lane with a screech of tyres.

We attend a patient in a dark apartment filled with cigarette smoke after that, a man who's 'not feeling normal'. John asks him to define 'normal'. He can't, and nor can we. The man gets a check-up all the same. Then we pick up a woman lying in a gutter, so drunk she's soiled herself. We cocoon her in a blanket with just her arm exposed for a drip, and give her some medicine to stop her from spewing. It's one less thing we'll have to mop out.

When the ambulance has been properly sanitised, we're sent to Taylor Square for a man at T2. It's a dance club where people can party for days, their eyes kept open by drugs and Red Bull. Our man complains that he's too tired to stand and wants to be carried.

'Been dancing since Friday,' he says with a groan.

But he's embarrassed to be leaving the club on a stretcher. John suggests he pull the bedsheet up over his head to hide his face from the queue outside.

Lying motionless and shrouded, our patient sparks momentary pandemonium in the line-up as we leave. It appears to the crowd that we're carting out a corpse.

'Oh my God!' shrieks a man, clutching his face in horror, as two girls start wailing. In no time at all, the queue has dispersed.

By 5 am, things have quietened down and the hordes of wasted punters have mostly drifted off, leaving a trail of fast-food junk and pools of vomit in their wake. It won't be long before an efficient team of cleaners wielding high-pressure hoses blitz the footpaths. By 7 am, there'll be little evidence left of the night's drunken carnage, as thousands of tourists leave fancy hotels with their cameras and bumbags, ready to explore this postcard-perfect city.

We don't see a soul on our return to the station. At this hour Bondi is more like a country town than Sydney's busiest beach, five minutes from the CBD. We've emerged from the city's underbelly and into the light. As a hint of pink dawn appears in the sky we think we're finally done.

But it's not to be. There's one last job to see us off. Up at The Gap, our second home.

While walking his dog, a man has found a pair of running shoes by the edge of the cliff. There's a car in the no-stopping zone too, keys in the ignition. It's a $300 ticket if you're caught in that spot. No one takes the risk unless they've decided they won't be around to pay the fine.

Our eyes are blinded by the sun heaving itself from the ocean. We squint against the glare, scanning for a body in the waves below. But there's only the gold of sunlight on water.

'Too hard to see,' I say.

'Might have gone under,' says a policeman who's arrived just behind us.

'Might never come up,' says John.

The air is fresh and clean and cool, the air of a new day. I inhale deep breaths the way Jerry does in the mornings, and with each one I feel the heaviness of my night lifting away.

CHAPTER 7

My mum and dad are worried about me. They call up in the morning to make sure I'm getting sleep, that I'm eating enough fruit, all the usual things. My mum reckons I sound depressed; her instincts are good, but I don't feel too bad. She drives over the bridge from Lane Cove after lunch. She wants to check on me in person and brings a casserole and my favourite ginger cake. She knows how miserable I get on my own. I'm sure she still remembers how badly I took breaking up with my first proper girlfriend at the age of eighteen. Back then I was so depressed I couldn't eat for a week. But that was before my chosen line of work gave me a suit of emotional armour.

Mum tidies my kitchen a bit and we have a cup of tea. She asks about Kaspia. I tell Mum I haven't seen her in a while but urge her not to worry.

'It's just a trial separation, a short break, that's all.' She's probably taking this harder than I am. Mothers often do. A while back she warned me not to take Kaspia for granted. She said, 'A relationship needs attention like a flower needs water.' And she knows about gardening; her garden is abundant. But I guess I didn't listen.

I tell her it's time I got ready for work. We hug and she leaves. Then I set up the ironing board to press my shirt and trousers.

My second night shift with John starts simply enough. A nursing-home patient with constipation, another with pneumonia.

The next one's a little trickier. I follow John up a flight of stairs to a top-floor apartment. The door is open and we find a man in a suit and tie sitting at a table eating his dinner with silver cutlery. His name is William, a retired doctor. We call out from a metre away, but he doesn't look up. William's wife, Margaret, has her back to the wall. She's visibly shaken. In a quivering voice she tells us that her husband, to whom she's been married for fifty years, has Alzheimer's and he's been rapidly going downhill. Within the past month his behaviour has become aggressive, violent even. On this occasion, according to Margaret, he pulled a carving knife from the kitchen drawer and held it to her throat. He threatened to kill her if she didn't cook him his favourite meal: steak and gravy with green beans and potato gems.

'But I didn't *have* any beans!' she cries.

John puts a comforting arm around her. Meanwhile I approach her husband, who continues chewing his steak as if we're not in the room.

'Excuse me, William,' I say, leaning down. 'We're paramedics from the ambulance service. Is everything okay?'

He must have heard, but he doesn't react.

'Your wife's called us because she's frightened. She says you threatened her with a knife.'

This time he stops eating and looks at us with irritation.

'Who the hell're you? What're ya talking about? I love my wife! We've been married fifty years. I'd never do that!'

'William!' his wife calls from the corner, her voice trembling. 'You said you'd *kill me* if I didn't give you beans. Don't you remember? You had a *knife*.'

He starts eating again and shakes his head. Through a mouthful of potato he grumbles, 'She's a crazy woman. Don't believe a word she says. Can't you see she's trying to get rid of me? After all that I've done for her. It's a bloody disgrace!'

By this time William's wife is crying loudly into John's shoulder. Framed black-and-white photos on the walls show them as a beautiful couple embracing on a park bench at Circular Quay, sometime in the fifties. In another they're standing on the deck of an ocean liner, dressed in loose whites for a Pacific cruise. Smaller pictures of children and grandchildren are propped up in rows. Laughing faces at barbecues and parties and graduations. As I move through their private exhibition and delve deeper into their history, I wonder at how tragic an end this is to such a meaningful relationship. I'm filled with pity as we finally convince the old doctor to come to hospital.

'Stupid cow,' he growls as we lead him out.

When I look back at Margaret and see her weeping in John's arms, I swear there are tears in John's eyes too.

An hour later, a twenty-one-year-old woman in Rose Bay calls us for a sore throat.

'Do you have a lozenge?' John asks her.

'A lozenge?'

'A lozenge. We don't stock them unfortunately. Do you have one?'

'Maybe. In the kitchen drawer.'

Our patient makes no effort to move from the bed. I wander into her kitchen and open her kitchen drawer and see a packet of Strepsils. I bring them back to John. With no detectable sarcasm he asks the woman, 'Would you like me to pop one in your mouth?'

'Yes please,' she replies.

It's only natural to be frustrated by inappropriate emergency calls. But at some point I realised this frustration never improved anything. It just made me feel lousy. In any case, the smallest ailment looms large for some people. They may not have the faculties to manage this stress, or to think of other options. They also don't know the wider consequences of their call. No one's told the woman with a sore throat that she's tying up the only available ambulance in a fifteen-kilometre radius. Or the woman last month who called us for pins and needles in her leg after her Labrador had slept on it.

'How's the lozenge?' John asks before we go.

'Good, thanks. I feel much better,' our patient replies.

We wish her a speedy recovery and drive away.

John tells me that he's almost used up his nightly 'quota of sympathy'. It's not even 9 pm.

'Two hours in, compassion level low,' he reports. That's when we get squeezed the hardest, of course.

The next address is all too familiar. It's the residence of two former nurses, a couple who've made an art of being unwell. They are, as one doctor at a local hospital put it, 'a pair of munchies'. In other words, sufferers of Munchausen syndrome, a condition in which people feign illness, disease or mental trauma to attract sympathy.

The man is well dressed and well read. He's articulate, and patronising. His wife is an actress par excellence. Both have years of experience nursing on general wards and know all about sickness: how it's done, what investigations and procedures ought to be conducted, what they're entitled to by law, the words required to get it, and how medical staff should behave. Their luxurious home, bought recently from money generated by another medical negligence settlement, is packed with physiology books and medical journals, up-to-date research on new and exciting illnesses. They are never simultaneously unwell; the roles of patient and caregiver swap from week to week.

When their varied medical complaints cause them pain, there will never be quite enough analgesia we can give them. They always want more, and running out of morphine from our kit is not uncommon, despite them having plenty of their own. They're on just about every pain reliever on the market and they have been separately admitted for opioid overdoses. Both are under sixty years of age, but each has a pill list longer than the average ninety-year-old. These pills are heaped in packets on their dining-room table, all from different doctors and pharmacies.

It's hard to know how to help this couple exploiting the health system for sympathy, drugs and money. If they fail to get attention they pen long letters of complaint and threaten lawsuits, several of which they've won.

John groans. 'Which one is it?'

Our data terminal says the patient is female.

'It's her,' I say.

'Her?'

'Her.'

John closes his eyes. 'No, no, no. Not her! I can't do it!'

He decides to use his 'wildcard'.

Some paramedics in the city have been using the informal wildcard system for years. No one knows who began it, but it goes like this: if the treating paramedic wants to get out of an unpleasant task, they can turn the job over to their partner by simply saying 'wildcard'. Problem is, in any given shift, the treating paramedic has just *one* wildcard to play. I, for instance, might use my wildcard for a vomiting patient. Vomit's not for me. Blood is fine. In such scenarios, I play the wildcard and my partner steps in. This wouldn't be so bad were it not for the fact that John can use a wildcard just as easily as I can. For this reason, not everyone likes the game.

We go in and the woman's on the ground with a painful knee, as she often is. She's on fentanyl patches and other powerful drugs, but still begs for morphine. We've been through it all before. Denying her request guarantees a complaint, and the time and stress involved in answering it and waiting for the outcome simply isn't worth it. While John sets up the stretcher I give her the morphine, and we carry her out. We don't mess around. Some of us call it a 'short back and sides'. In and out, load and go. It's the best approach for critical patients as much as it is for calls near the end of our shift, or for patients we want to spend as little time as possible with.

Christmas parties are going on all over the place and the city streets are swarming. Ladies teeter on high heels and men in groups slap one another with excitement. Some women in a car at the lights flash their boobs at John.

'Oh God,' says John in camp disgust. 'And they think they just did me a favour . . .'

Cruising through Kings Cross is a great diversion for John. He loves people-watching, like I do. But his caustic commentary on some of the passing punters seems more vicious tonight, given his current state. It's like he's revolted by all that used to amuse him. At Bayswater Road he nods at a young woman crossing in front of us who's wearing a pair of cut-off shorts with pockets hanging out the front.

'Can you believe girls wear those things?' he says.

'Not a good look.'

'It's a fucked look, that's what it is. A fucked look in a fucked world.'

Across the street a pack of young men push each other round and one of them trips over, spilling hot chips. A passing vagrant drops to his knees and eats them out of the gutter. There's a row of Harley-Davidsons and bikies in their colours leaning against them, smoking. Neon flashes above the awnings and thudding techno pulses from a nearby club, where the line to get in snakes around the block.

'Fucking queues,' says John. 'These people queue for an hour to get in, then queue for an hour to reach the bar, then queue for an hour to use the toilet.'

I tell him he's sounding old. I'm pretty sure he spent his youth in bars like that.

Control are calling us for a job on Bayswater Road, an unconscious girl. She's only eighteen and her friends are convinced that her drink has been spiked. It's a common complaint these days, but genuine spikings are rare.

John isn't holding his famous acid tongue tonight. 'Which of her twenty drinks was spiked, then?' he asks her teenage friends. I'm relieved his sardonic humour is lost on the group. One of her friends even answers, 'Who knows?'

After dropping her to Sydney Hospital we drive down Ward Avenue, where the streetlights are out, and see a solitary man in a trench coat waving frantically. I pull up and wind down the window.

'Sir, you all right?'

He says, 'I'm losing control of myself.'

'How so?'

'I'm developing homelessness.'

'Developing?'

I'm curious about his use of words, as if being homeless was an illness. I guess it could happen like that. You lose your job, hit the bottle, can't pay rent, get evicted, crash on a friend's lounge, get kicked off that, then walk around and end up asleep in a doorway. Or, as one man once described it to me, 'start camping in the city'.

'Last week I wasn't so bad,' the man says. 'I did some window-washing, had spare change, bought some milk and cereal, cut a banana on top. I was in a hostel, it was pretty good. But this week's gone to shit and I'm back on the street.'

'What's for breakfast now?' asks John.

'Whatever I find,' says the man.

We drop him at hospital to see a social worker. Afterwards John says, 'Could've been me, that guy, you know.' And I remember his comment about Missionbeat.

He says, 'I was thinking about a spot in Woolloomooloo under the railway bridge. I've had my eye on it. I don't mind the tramps down there. You can find some quality half-eaten food in bins these days; you'd be surprised.'

'If you eat hospital sandwiches you'll eat anything,' I say.

I'm glad Mick came through with a unit for John to stay in. But it's only temporary. What happens next month, when Mick gets a full-paying tenant?

'Why don't you find your own place like I did?' I ask him.

'And seal my fate?' he replies. 'You need to stop pretending you'll get your girl back.'

My heart sinks and I feel defensive. He knows less about Kaspia and me than I know about him and Antonio. We're friends as well as colleagues and we have a close bond, yet we're also private people who don't talk very much about life outside work. Most of us at Bondi Station are good at keeping work and home life separate. I know he's been with Antonio roughly as long as I've been with Kaspia, but every relationship and every separation is different. It's not getting an apartment on your own that seals your fate. It's the loss of hope for a reconciliation that does it.

Victor, one of our regular psychiatric patients, has been drinking again. His girlfriend usually calls us, fearing for her life. Victor turns violent quickly and sometimes needs restraining. This is not an easy task. He reckons he's a former Israeli Defense Forces commando who once 'killed hundreds of Arabs in their sleep'. I used to think it was a grandiose delusion. But once I got to know Victor I started to suspect his IDF story might actually be true.

We ascend the stairs of his Housing Commission block cautiously, remembering last week down in Little Bay, the man and his cricket bat. I tell John we should wait for the cops, but he keeps going. Of late he's been more reckless than usual.

John raps on the door. We both stand to the side, a habit of situational awareness we're not even conscious of. We shouldn't be doing this, not without cops, not with Victor.

Victor's girlfriend opens up and I follow John in. The alcohol fumes in the unit are potent. Victor's in the lounge room, wearing nothing but underpants. In his hands are two long knives, their blades pointed down. When he sees us he begins to swish them about like he's some kind of ninja, spitting and grunting and growling in anger. I scan the room then try to retreat the way we entered. But Victor's girlfriend stands in the doorway.

'Help him!' she orders, hands on her hips.

I feel for the button on my portable radio, the duress alarm. As I push it for the second time in less than a fortnight I trust the system is working, that the number is logged, that alarms will go off in our distant control room, that police will be sent.

'Settle down, Victor. You know what'll happen if police see all this,' says John.

But Victor dances closer, waving his knives, his eyes wide and mad. He likes to remind us he's a ruthless assassin, but it's the first time we've seen him with knives.

He moves to within an arm's length of John, but John stands his ground, hands raised in defence.

'John!' I yell urgently, my call to retreat. I want to run but won't leave my partner, and he still isn't budging. Has he lost all common sense?

A door bangs open behind me, the door to the street. Police pile into the room and John steps back. A sergeant points a taser, yelling, 'Put the knives down, Victor. Put them down, or I'll shoot!'

But Victor ignores him, keeps on with his antics.

'We're here to help you. Drop the knives!'

Victor growls again, then lunges for the sergeant. The cop pulls the trigger. The double barbs fly out and pierce Victor's chest. A charge hits the cables and he drops to the floor.

His girlfriend starts to shriek and curse in horror. A moment ago she begged us for protection. Now she pounces on the sergeant, grabs him round the neck, punches at his head. She's dragged off by the others and handcuffed on the ground.

After I watch Victor and his girlfriend being taken away I go back inside. John's still there, frozen in thought. Why didn't he leave when he had the chance? We could have been knifed; he must have known that. But he's not at his best and I choose to say nothing; a lecture's the last thing he needs right now, I'm sure.

It's 3 am and we're parked on the corner of Oxford and Palmer. We watch the drunks stumble in the gutters, clutching pizzas, waiting for taxis. A young punter knocks on my window, while two of his friends snigger behind him.

I wind down my window just a few inches.

'Mate,' says the guy, 'can you breathalyse me? I need to prove to those bouncers that I'm not really drunk.'

'Fucking idiot,' John says, loud enough for the guy to hear. I put up the window and shut the world out again.

When another man knocks a few minutes later I try to ignore him. But then I see that it's Raymond, a friend of a friend who thinks he's a gangster. He wears ghetto fashions: an oversized T-shirt that looks like a nightie and a big baseball cap. But his best accessory is a stainless-steel grill that he clips to his teeth. Last year he turned up at a Sugartime afterparty, tried selling cocaine. I asked him to leave, politely of course. And here he is now. What does he want?

'Hey Ben, yo!' he says, flashing his grill. I open the window and he reaches inside to shake my hand. John looks at him suspiciously.

Raymond laughs. 'You boys waitin' for a dude to get whacked?'

I say, 'Raymond, meet John. John, meet Raymond.'

'Yo,' Raymond says, nodding at John. He glances around, then leans through the window. 'You want some Armani? Suits I'm talkin', I've got thirty. Need to offload 'em. Gotta do it right now, know what I mean? Rock-bottom dollar. Genuine product. Cool if it's no, yo. How about candy? Candy-cane maybe? To get through the night? How about that?'

John's eyes light up now.

'Gold dust? Pepsi cola? Know what I mean?'

'How much?' asks John.

I look at my partner and see he's not joking.

'For you boys, cost price, yo.'

John takes out his wallet, looking for money.

We're out in the open on a Darlinghurst corner with hundreds of punters milling around, not to mention the cops I can see on patrol. So I tell Raymond, 'All good, mate. See you round, eh?'

'No sweat, yo,' he says. 'Take it easy now, boys.'

John starts up the ambulance, does a U-turn up Oxford. 'Where'd you find him?'

Before I can reply, the radio cuts in and we're given a case.

'I want Raymond's number,' John demands. 'Understand me?'

Then he flicks on the siren and goes through a red.

Our last patient tonight is a man with angina, a welcome relief from the drunks and assaults. Ron is seventy, a retired police sergeant. He is friendly and chatty on the way to St Vinnies. It's 3.30 am and I warn him about how wild it can be at the hospital. But he knows about that. He worked at Rose Bay as a cop in the eighties. I ask if The Gap was busy then too. The question throws him off kilter and his smile fades away.

Ron closes his eyes, says, 'That place gives me nightmares. It's always been bad. The Gap made me quit. One day I just walked and never came back.'

'What happened?'

'A fuck-up, that's what. A guy on the edge who wanted to jump and was there for two hours, driving us nuts. He was wasting our time, and I told him directly, if he wanted to jump he should bloody get on with it. And that's what he did. The guy bloody jumped. Those were the days before we knew about counselling. I said the wrong thing and I've carried the burden.'

Our monitor's beeping as Ron's heart rate goes up. He puts his hand to his chest. It's time to change the subject.

Negotiating with someone at The Gap is all very well if they have a change of heart and come back from the edge. But if it goes the other way, what then? I'm grateful it's never happened to me, although it could any day. The mind of a person standing on the edge is a slowly ticking time bomb that we try to defuse before it's too late. A few careless words are like cutting the wrong wire.

We stop for the sunrise on the way back to Bondi station. We park at the north end of the beach and take in the view.

'What if things start improving with you and Antonio, now you've moved out?'

'Move out and it's over, I told you before.'

We sit there in silence, the sun on our faces.

Time apart is important; it offers space for reflection, realisation and progress. Even the counsellor Kaspia and I saw together told us that separation helps 'maintain our identity'. Moving out is not the end. It might have the opposite effect, might refresh the relationship. At least, I tell myself that.

Surf lifesaving veterans, their speedos printed with BONDI, walk slowly up the ramp, dripping from an early swim. They smile and give us a wave, oblivious to the night we've had. Japanese tourists in sun-visor caps line up their slippers in neat rows before testing the sand with their toes.

John points to the clifftops.

'Albatross – see it?'

The bird is a beauty. It rides on the currents of air for a while then, spying a fish in the blue depths below, plummets like a missile and pierces the sea.

'Ever wish you'd been born as a bird?' John asks.

The albatross rises above the surface again, wings laden with water.

'Yeah, sometimes,' I say. 'What about you?'

'All the time,' he replies.

CHAPTER 8

Christmas is only one week away. I go to Bronte on my second day off and park on Pacific Street outside the apartment block Kaspia and I used to live in. I loved this place. It was a charmed life we had together, despite the arguments. I take a short cut to the beach down the side of the block, just as I did every day when we lived here.

The surf is no good so I throw out a blanket, read a book in the sun. I keep looking around to see if Kaspia's here but remember it's Thursday, a day she's at work.

The beach is deserted. It's different on weekends, but weekends don't mean much with the odd hours we work; penalty rates, maybe. That's about it. Sometimes I feel I must look indulgent, surfing or relaxing at the beach on a weekday. It's the way I come down from the adrenalin of work. But people might wonder what million-dollar business has allowed me such leisure. Or perhaps they imagine I'm an unemployed bum.

No wonder paramedics' relationships can be troubled. We work while others play and play while others work. Days off in the week might be calm in the suburbs, and the parks may be empty, galleries uncrowded, but we end up on our own in the middle of the week while our partners are alone on weekends, surrounded by couples and families.

My manager calls me while I'm still at the beach to offer me a day shift tomorrow. It's overtime rates, at Paddington station.

I'll be teamed up with Tracy, a vivacious, young ambo new in the job. She's awfully nice; too sweet, some have said. She's got rosy red cheeks and her blonde hair is braided with ribbons. She looks far too innocent for ambulance work, but in reality she's been on the road for months, so it's doubtful she has any innocence left. It doesn't take long for rookies like her to grow the thick skin they need to survive.

We're sent to a drowning at Elizabeth Bay. A man saw his neighbour fall into her pool. Tracy usually drives like a nana, but today she's on fire and we get there in no time. A man waves us down.

'Go ahead,' Tracy says, 'I'll follow with the gear.'

Running is a no-no. It makes people panic. You might lose your footing, fall over, get hurt, and if you *do* reach your patient you'll end up too breathless to be of any use. But I make an exception. I run up the side path, hurdle a gate and land with a stumble. I look up and I see her, an elderly woman, facedown in the pool, her nightie ballooning around her in the water.

I pull off my boots and whip off my shirt, then I jump into the shallows, half-swimming, half-wading. I grab the patient's shoulder, roll her over. She's in her late seventies, her face pale and slack-jawed. To me she looks dead, but I drag her out and drain her airway.

Tracy arrives, lugging equipment. I'm waist deep in water as we work on the woman. Tracy does the compressions and I ask how she managed to open the gate. She giggles a little, as she pumps up and down, and tells me she simply lifted the latch.

Another crew turns up and we all work together. We continue our efforts while loading the patient onto our stretcher. Then we drive her to St Vinnies, doing CPR in the back. I do compressions with one hand, while holding on to a bar for support with the other, as the ambulance bounces over median strips and gutters. CPR in a moving vehicle isn't that effective, but we're committed now. After reaching the hospital, the senior doctor calls time of death a minute later. It's another anticlimax I can add to the list.

I'm used to that feeling, the deflation I get after cardiac arrests. Even though so few of them make it, our monthly newsletter is full of survivors, photos of those who've returned from the dead. They're sometimes presented with little heart badges, trophies or watches, supplied by the company that makes our defibrillators. Everyone's smiling: the patient, the families, the brave paramedics, those who can say they finally saved one. And the ambos look happier than the people they've saved. One day I might also appear in a photo, presenting a patient with a near-death memento. But with my luck it's doubtful.

We return to the station. Tracy thanks me for making the rescue. She tells me she's thinking of starting a club with a group of her girlfriends, a paramedic women's club that will meet once a month to talk about other careers.

'The Society of Ladies, we'll call it,' she says. 'We'll chat about dream jobs: the life of a florist or how to run a pet shop, that kind of thing.'

She's been here five minutes and is already plotting escape. For me it was different. As a brand-new recruit I was keen for the action, the trauma, the drama. I sat near the radio waiting for a call; I couldn't get enough. I dreamt about jumping into swimming pools with my trousers still on to save unconscious women.

'We'll meet wearing dresses and bitch about uniforms,' Tracy tells me as we drive.

Maybe to keep our nightmares at bay, all we need is high tea: some scones and cream and a cup of Earl Grey.

After I've put on a dry pair of pants, we head to Waterloo for a man who's experiencing psychosis. His apartment is decorated with pages he's torn from pornographic magazines, framed and hung up. One centrefold model holds a mean-looking dog and a bundle of chains. Our patient has stars tattooed on his face, and when I lift up his shirtsleeve to take a BP I see another tatt of a woman with her legs spread wide.

There's a *pssssst* sound above us and a wall-mounted air-freshener shoots a spray of lavender mist over our heads. As the synthetic fragrance enters my lungs I begin to feel giddy.

'Let's get out of here,' I tell Tracy.

When we walk the guy out he says he hasn't slept in a week, says he feels like 'killing someone – anyone will do'. Tracy's glad she's not sitting in the back with him. I do my best to keep the guy calm with friendly smiles and conversation.

When I ask his date of birth for my paperwork, I see that today is his birthday.

'Happy birthday!' I say, then call out to Tracy, 'It's our patient's birthday! Shall we find a cake shop on the way to hospital?' We do these things from time to time, and we're not the only ones. The other night we saw an ambulance outside Ben & Jerry's, picking up ice cream for their patient with schizophrenia. Whatever it takes to keep our patients happy is a good thing in my books. It's also a matter of safety. We're confined in the back of an ambulance a foot away from people who are often agitated and unpredictable. It should be in our protocol to buy them cake and ice cream, if that is what's required.

Before Tracy can answer me the patient grunts that he's a diabetic and 'can't have fucken cake'. He drops his head and looks like he's about to cry.

A lady in her eighties leads us down a concrete path lined with pruned rosebushes to a house that smells like gingerbread. 'My son, he not wake up,' she says in a southern European accent.

A man lies prone in a bathroom. He's half-in, half-out of the shower recess, in his left hand a drained bottle of gin. Empty pill packets are scattered around. Tracy goes out to get the stretcher. Then I see that our patient is Hamish, a paramedic from a neighbouring station. Only a few months ago we worked a shift together and he seemed to be fine, if a little subdued. Lately I've heard he's been having some issues: depression, delusions, addiction. The service had recently stood him down while deciding if he was fit for the job.

'Hamish!' I shout, shaking his shoulder. He's wearing a polo shirt embroidered with our ambulance logo, and his feet are laced into rescue boots. A stethoscope and glove pouch lie in the sink and a fluorescent ambulance jacket hangs on a hook. I suspect the items have been placed there intentionally, symbols of his beloved profession now under threat, or to make sure we know that he's one of us.

Hamish groans through the oxygen mask I've attached to his face. Tracy wheels our stretcher down the hall towards me.

'It's Hamish,' I tell her.

Tracy turns pale.

I nod. 'Polypharmacy, with alcohol, GCS twelve. Can you drop the bed to half-height? Reckon we can drag him onto it.'

As we head to Prince of Wales we phone our supervisor. We don't have a choice. Tracy and I promise each other we'll keep the matter quiet, but a semiconscious paramedic in the resuscitation bay at Emergency doesn't stay secret for long. By midday there won't be a medic in the city who won't know about Hamish.

There've been many worse cases of paramedics called to their own. Hamish won't die from his overdose today. But six paramedics I've worked with have ended their lives. Death is demystified to us; it's the business we're in. We know what works and what doesn't. We understand anatomy, physiology, pharmacology. And those of us with their hearts set on suicide will rarely survive.

*

Tracy and I are both a little shaken after helping Hamish. The time is right for a treat to cheer us up. We see a Turkish takeaway joint and Tracy tells me how much she loves baklava. I pull over and reverse the ambulance back to the shop. We buy a few slices, but get a call before we can eat them. Not that it's an obstacle to us; while I hurtle along with lights and sirens blaring, Tracy leans over and gives me a bite of baklava. This might appear intimate to others, but there's nothing romantic about it. We're just a brother and sister of the paramedic family, and I hate a sticky steering wheel.

Many husbands and wives of paramedics struggle to grasp this platonic relationship. Even Kaspia's had her moments. But witnessing all manner of tragedies together inevitably builds a bond. Paramedics share pain and conflict, suffering and death. Like soldiers who've fought side by side, we're united forever by what we have seen. In that sense we understand each other, at least a *facet* of each other, much better than our non-paramedic partners ever can.

High on sugary baklava, we arrive at a familiar housing block in Redfern. On level twelve our caller takes a good minute to unlock his door. There's a CCTV camera on the opposite wall, red light flashing. A man in his thirties with wild eyes opens the door. He wants to know if we're with the FBI. We shake our heads. CIA? No.

The man lets us in and tells us his place is bugged. Inside are a dozen cameras. He knows secrets – state secrets, explosive secrets – he says, and he's being monitored. It looks more like he's monitoring himself. We know he suffers schizophrenia and Tracy asks if he's taking his medication. He says he ran out a few days ago. He agrees to come to hospital after we tell him he'll be safe there. The man is paranoid and delusional; that's our assumption. But I often have to wonder: what if some of these patients are telling the truth? What if they really *are* being watched, if they really *do* have state secrets? Nothing surprises me anymore.

An hour later we scream down Anzac Parade to a woman having a heart attack. We turn into a peaceful suburban back-street, ditch our siren and skid into the gutter. On the verandah of a red-brick house we see a wizened man on a rocking chair who looks like he's been sitting there for decades.

We exit the ambulance and go through the gate. I open the old man's door thinking we're here for his wife.

'Is the patient inside?' I enquire.

But he shakes his head.

'No?' I ask. 'So where, then?'

He shakes his head again; he's a man of few words. Then it dawns on me we're at the wrong house.

'Did you call for an ambulance?'

Again he shakes his head.

Before we can leave we hear a loud barking and a sausage dog charges right through the door and jumps on my leg. The old man ignores it. He doesn't look over, doesn't call the dog to heel. He just sits there indifferently and watches me curse and try to shake the thing off. Tracy picks up the kits and heads to the wagon. I finally manage to send the dog flying then leap down the stairs. But the dog's on my tail, chasing me over the lawn, yapping like mad. With seconds to spare I exit the gate and slam it behind me.

When we reach the right address, a woman in her eighties with chest pain says her name is Nana Cat. It's not hard to see why. There's a cat on her shoulder and four in her lap. She tells us her chest pains came on after walking to the shops and back. Her complexion is grey and sweaty. If she wasn't so sick I'd be patting her cats. Dogs might not like me, but cats I get on with.

Tracy readies the oxygen while I wheel in the stretcher as close as I can. I drop it to half-height a metre away. The patient will only need two little steps to be on it. Don't walk a chest pain, I was told in my training, but it's a couple of steps, hardly a strain.

We slowly help Nana Cat to her feet. Her fingers are cold and an icy chill passes from her hands to mine, then right up my arms and down through my spine. My whole body shivers and I get a bad feeling in the pit of my stomach. Never did I imagine two little steps could be so much effort. She can barely take one, let alone two. And as she tries for her second, she stops in her tracks. Her mouth gapes open and closed, like that of a fish out of water. All remaining colour drains from her face.

I scoop her legs from under her and lay her on the stretcher. She looks up at me and we lock eyes. Her look is screaming what her voice cannot. Her eyes are burning with fear, and the realisation that these are her final seconds on earth before a death she hasn't prepared for.

Tracy calls for backup.

I pull out my scissors.

'Set up the defib,' I say, still holding Nana Cat's gaze. A second later her eyes lose their panic. She looks over my shoulder, to a place beyond the room, somewhere both close and far away. Her fingers relax in my grip and she submits to her fate. Before she dies she lifts her right hand in the air, as if reaching for something beautiful. The look on her face is now one of wonder, like she's discovered how to fly. Then her pupils dilate and fog over.

Her pulse is gone before she loses consciousness.

'CPR,' I tell Tracy, and she starts compressions.

My trauma shears cut through Nana Cat's blouse. I pull out the defib pads, peel them off and stick them on.

The monitor shows VF: ventricular fibrillation.

'Charging up,' I say. 'Going for a shock. Stand clear!'

We defibrillate. Her body spasms but she doesn't respond.

Another ambulance is coming. I cannulate and draw up adrenalin, then go for another shock. When the other crew arrives we continue our efforts. We get a heartbeat back and put Nana Cat in the ambulance, but she loses her pulse again soon after that.

When we reach the hospital the doctor seems annoyed. With a sigh he asks, 'How long has she been down for? What's the history?' He's looking for a reason to stop resuscitation, he thinks it's no use.

As the doctor listens he gives a casual wave for a female medical student to 'have a go at CPR'. I step back from Nana Cat's chest. The medical student takes over but her compressions are weak. I want to push her aside and jump on again, do the job properly. But our role as paramedics ends right here.

A few minutes later the doctor looks around and asks, 'Everybody happy?'

No one says a thing.

Then he glances at the wall clock and declares the time of death.

I bite my lip. I should have piped up, said no, I *wasn't* happy. This shouldn't be the way to end resuscitation. In the case of Nana Cat I know my objectivity is tainted by having seen her alive, by the fact we watched her breathe her last. Not to mention the guilt I now feel about walking her to the stretcher. Could those two little steps have sealed her demise?

'Just bad luck,' the doctor says as he leaves the resus bay, peeling off his gloves. 'We spend a lifetime abusing our hearts. Eventually it catches up with us.'

Outside, Tracy is sitting on the back step of the ambulance with her head in her hands. I phone the control room and ask for time out. They give it reluctantly, and I understand why. They routinely have emergencies waiting. I say we won't be long. We drive down to Coogee and order hot chocolates and sit by the beach. We watch as an afternoon storm rumbles in.

It's easy to see that Tracy's shaken up. I put my hand on her shoulder. When I started in the job a manager once told me, 'If you can't stand the heat, get out of the kitchen.' Now we get offered professional help from a counselling service, but only when we want it, which isn't very often. Most of us would rather hang out at the beach chatting informally with each other, drinking hot chocolate.

This is not the first time a patient has died on me, but Nana Cat is the first one to have looked in my eyes at the moment of death. What's most disturbing is knowing that I was the final image she saw. When I come to breathe my last, I hope to be looking at the people I love or the wide, open sea or tall, snowy mountains. Not the sweaty face of a hapless paramedic.

CHAPTER 9

On my first day back for my regular shifts John turns up late and looks like a tramp, his uniform unironed. Once we've got the ambulance ready he goes straight to the lounge and lies down.

At 7.30 am he's compelled to get up when we're given a case. From his look and his smell, I suspect he's at work to stop himself drinking. I ask him how he's going, what's new with Antonio. He just quietly shakes his head.

On the balcony of a unit block a shirtless man with a hairy chest is lifting dumbbells. Seeing us below, he stops and yells out, 'Take that bastard away!'

We find our patient in the folds of a torn-up lounge chair. It seems he hasn't showered in weeks. The room stinks of sweat, old beer and cigarette butts, with the whiff of charred meat. It's a smell we all recognise, the odour of neglect. His body is little more than dry skin around a skeleton. Faded tattoos of swallows and daggers adorn both his arms. There's a bottle of sherry on the table and a cigarette burning between his tar-stained fingers. His eyes stare vacantly at the television set until John switches it off. John hates it when people call us but keep watching TV while we're standing there to help.

'Merry Christmas,' says John, in a monotone.

'It's Christmas?' asks the man.

'Any minute now, yes. I'm John. What's your name?'

'Bob.'

'What can we do for you, Bob?'

'Been depressed,' he replies.

'And you called yourself an ambulance?'

John's not always like this. His sympathy for patients, and his tenderness, are well known. But these past few months he's been different. The John I'm seeing is more often impatient, intolerant, jaded. His humour is shifting from cheeky to sardonic. His compassion is dwindling, a classic sign of burnout in the realm of first responders.

'Yeah, I called you,' says Bob, glaring at John. 'Got a problem with that? You ever been depressed?'

'Matter of fact, yes. But I never called an ambulance. Anyway, how long have you been feeling this way?'

'Whole damn week. Come to think of it, the whole bloody year. Actually, I've been depressed from the day I was born. Even as a baby I tried killing myself.'

What an odd thing to say.

'You live here alone?' asks John.

'Yeah.'

'Ever been married?'

'No.' Bob pauses for a moment. 'Had a girlfriend once, a long time ago.'

His sunken eyes search in the distance for memories. I wait for the glimmer of a smile, but there's nothing. I've met old men like Bob a hundred times before. They live alone or out on the streets, their stories too familiar. A long-lost love, the one that got away, or walked away, or cheated on them and disappeared, or died an early death. The one they loved above all, who can never be replaced. Our city is full of lonely men who've locked themselves away or carry broken hearts from doorway to doorway.

Looking at John as he drives us back to hospital, I wonder if he's thinking the same thoughts I am. His face is taut, a dam holding back an impossible pressure. I imagine he's reflecting on the simple mistakes that spell the end for lovers, mistakes that can make them feel more dead than alive.

*

After dropping Bob off we're dispatched to a woman hit by a car a block from St Vinnies. Her shopping is lying all over the road. She's confused and combative and writhing around. We suspect she's suffered a haemorrhage in her brain. Her life's on the line, so we load her up quickly. It's a race against time and John does what he can in the back of the ambulance as I floor it to hospital. The trip is all over in less than eight minutes. She goes into neurosurgery. Her chances are good.

It's been a busy start to our shift. We drive to North Bondi and pull up in the car park to watch the swell come in. The ocean is a healer; its effect is calming and it helps us gain perspective. Shame John and I get so little time this morning. But even a glimpse of the water works wonders.

Bondi 402, you on the air? 402?

Affirmative. Go ahead.

Got one down in Bondi for you.

We start up the engine and proceed to a blond-brick unit block two streets from the beach. A woman yells, 'Hang – I want to hang! Let me hang!'

A crowd of young backpackers and locals has gathered on a nature strip. They point to an apartment high up, where they reckon an old Chinese woman and her husband reside.

John and I make our way down a path to the entrance. We don't get far. A glass bottle whistles past and clears John's head by an inch, shattering on the concrete beside us. We both duck in time to avoid a vase, closely followed by a set of dinner plates, hurled from an open window. Smashed porcelain lies everywhere. It's not the first time this fortnight we've been attacked. But this time, thankfully, John retreats to the street. We wait for the police.

Things could be worse, I say to John. At least we're not the target of a sniper. Getting shot at is a real danger for paramedics in other countries I've been to, like Mexico, South Africa and Pakistan. Jam jars and china we can handle.

A police cage truck pulls up at the very moment a wild-eyed woman begins crawling on all fours from the front of the building. She's wearing a gingham apron and her hair sticks up like she's been electrocuted. She's not let up her desperate screaming for a second. 'Hang! Hang! Let me hang!' She spits and snarls, contorting her face, before plonking herself cross-legged on the roadside. We watch with the crowd as she takes a cigarette case from the pocket of her apron and lights up a smoke. With a cigarette clamped between her teeth she begins her crawl again, this time across the street, growling like a wildcat. Police direct traffic around her.

'If we take her in the ambulance she'll tear it apart,' John says to the sergeant.

The conveyance of psychiatric patients is mostly done by ambulance because their problems are a health matter rather than a criminal one. Occasionally, though, when the patient's so violent they're a danger to us, we'll opt for a police truck to take them instead.

The sergeant nods and orders his officers to don leather gloves. He tells the patient she's under a schedule, a legal document that allows a mentally disturbed person to be apprehended against their will for transport to hospital. The police then pick up the woman, who's kicking and screaming, and put her in their wagon, locking the door behind her.

'We'll follow you in the ambulance,' I tell them.

Before we leave, one of the constables mentions to us that a man went off The Gap this morning.

'We almost called you,' he says, 'but there was nothing to do. Can you believe he flew up from Melbourne on the first Virgin flight of the day? Took a taxi to The Gap and over he went.'

'Ridiculous,' John says. 'If it was *my* last flight, I'd want to go Qantas.'

The cops have a chuckle, then catch themselves and get serious again. There's still a crowd watching and perceptions are everything. They can't have people thinking they're laughing at the woman in the police truck. By now she's settled down with her cursing, and she's no longer pounding on the back of the door either.

'Thank God,' says a cop. 'Peace and quiet.'

'Must have worn herself out,' says another.

Before the police pull away I decide to take a quick look through the small perspex window in the side of their truck.

The window is foggy, and a bit scratched up. But I see the lady clearly enough: she's lying unconscious, with her apron string tied around her neck.

'Shit!' I yell. 'Open it – she's strangled herself!'

The cops unbolt the door and drag the woman out. She's limp and comatose and frothing at the mouth. John pulls the stretcher from the ambulance and we heave our patient onto it. I toss our keys to one of the cops.

'Drive for us, will you?'

The cop nods and jumps in the front. The engine roars.

John ventilates the woman while I set up the monitor and look for a vein. 'Why is everyone necking themselves?' asks John. 'What the fuck's going on?'

By the time we reach the hospital the patient is awake again, and markedly calmer. But John's about ready to call it a day.

We've got less than thirty minutes to clean up, finish paperwork, go to the toilet, have a drink and prepare for the next emergency call. Sometimes they come in before we're ready. Ten minutes after arriving at St Vinnies I hear about a cardiac arrest in Surry Hills. No ambulance is available to respond, so I answer the radio and take the job. John makes a lame attempt to snatch the handset off me.

'What the hell are you doing?' he asks.

I shrug. 'There's no one else.'

'You're jumping a cardiac arrest? After the day we've had so far? You really think I want to work up a sweat pumping on somebody's chest, mess up our gear and carry some overweight bloke down a long flight of stairs?'

There aren't many cases I'll volunteer for. But life-threatening ones – the chokings, arterial bleeds, cardiac arrests, the ones where seconds count – those I'll take. I might have doubts that I've ever saved a life, but somewhere deep down I hang on to hope. Why else would I volunteer for this cardiac arrest if I didn't believe my luck might change, if this could be the one?

John's cranky. And he's right, I should've asked first.

'Sorry mate,' I say.

We drive to the address, our lights and siren scattering the lunch crowd. It's a ground-floor apartment, and we walk in to see a toothless man doing CPR on his friend. It was heroin, he tells us, panting as he pumps. We connect the defibrillator and find the patient in asystole, where the heart has lost all electrical activity. Not many will come back from that.

We take over resus and the patient's mate goes to sit on the lounge. He leans over a coffee table and starts eating a meat pie with a knife and fork.

'Came home and found him,' he says with his mouth full.

The man continues eating while we try to revive his friend. He stops only once, to loudly squirt ketchup onto his plate.

'Shit!' he says. 'Why does it always shoot out like that? Tomato fucking sauce.'

He starts eating again, loud enough to hear above the siren of our approaching backup ambulance.

'Fellas,' he says, 'do ya think he'll be able to stay here tonight? If he's staying, I'll put a pie in the oven for him.'

We don't get a chance to answer before a second crew from Redfern comes through the door. One of the paramedics, Andy, is quite the mischievous operator. The first thing he does is go to the stereo and hit the play button. The song 'If I Could Turn Back Time' comes on.

'Always curious about the music a person was listening to when they dropped,' says Andy, an intensive-care paramedic, rolling out his intubation kit. 'Everything seems to go better if a good tune is playing, don't you think?'

'Have you seen the costume Cher's wearing in the music video?' asks John, starting an IV. 'Fishnet body stocking over a one-piece swimsuit.'

The job goes smoothly enough. John runs the meds, Andy gets the tube, his partner does CPR, I work the defib. But after twenty minutes our patient is still in a flatline. We decide to wrap things up. I turn down the stereo volume slowly, a gentle fade-out, like a DJ. Then Andy looks at his watch and announces a time of death. The man's friend licks his plate and sits back on the lounge, holding his belly. With a lazy eye he sees us start to pack away our stuff.

'Dead?' he asks.

I nod. 'Yeah, mate. I'm sorry.'

'Well I fucken told him, didn't I. Nigel, I said, don't be shooting up on your own. It's not fucken worth it, I said. So what does he do?'

The man gets off the lounge and dumps his plate in the sink.

'The police are on their way,' Andy tells him. 'It's procedure, a matter for the coroner.'

'Nigel, Nigel, Nigel. Fucken idiot Nigel.' The man shakes his head. Then he takes a second pie and puts it in the oven. 'One thing's for sure though, mate. If ya gunna fucken die, someone else'll eat ya pie.'

Between jobs I get a phone call from my mother with the news that my youngest brother, Mark, a pilot, has saved a life. She reckons he dragged a bloke from the surf yesterday morning and revived him on the beach.

The story is hard to believe, so I call up Mark and catch him as he's getting ready to go out with his mates. He sounds distracted.

'Heard you saved a guy,' I say.

'Oh yeah, that.'

'Elaborate?'

Mark tells me he was waiting for a wave at Dee Why when a man surfing nearby rolled off his board and was facedown in the water. Mark swam over and grabbed him round the chest and swam the guy to shore, dragging his lifeless body up the beach. Along with a passing doctor and another surfer, he performed CPR for ten or so minutes. A bystander called an ambulance and ran to the surf club to get a defibrillator.

'By the time ambos got there the guy was coughing up sea water and trying to talk,' says Mark.

Hearing my brother recount his tale triggers weird emotions in me. Cynicism, doubt, jealousy, frustration. Shouldn't I be pleased for him? Proud of his achievement?

A nervous laugh escapes me and I say, 'Good on you, mate,' and remind him just how remarkable his saving of a life really is. The man would be dead now if not for him.

Mark says, 'Thanks, mate. Gotta go, we're about to hit the town.' He's way too dismissive for my liking. Too flippant. Does he grasp how significant and rare his save has been? I wish it was me who'd swum the guy in, done CPR. Mark saved a man but shrugs it off like it's nothing. How strange that a full-time paramedic like me can't safely say he's saved someone whose heart has stopped while my brother, a pilot, raises the dead on a sunny day off.

When I recount the story to John he says, 'To save them you have to be there on the spot, right when it happens.' But I know that already. It's a truth rarely spoken. Research has told us that for every minute without defibrillation, the chance of survival for a cardiac-arrest victim decreases by roughly ten per cent. A response time of ten minutes might not sound that bad, but for cardiac arrests it doesn't bode well. Maybe I need to drive faster.

Heavy clouds loom in the distance and it looks like one of those late summer storms. As the sun is snuffed out, we're sent to our third suicide attempt of the day, once again at The Gap. It's at Lighthouse Reserve, not quite Gap proper, but close enough to count.

'I've had enough of this. Just drop me at the Junction,' John says.

'You know I can't do that,' I reply.

'Say I'm sick, I've got the shits.'

'They're not stupid.'

'They'll find another car.'

'Can't do it, sorry.'

John purses his lips and crosses his arms as I step on the accelerator up Old South Head Road.

'Well *you* can do the talking, then,' he says. 'Consider it my wildcard. I'm staying in the car.'

I'll do it, I don't mind. I've seen John talk down dozens of people. He's one of the best, he's got nothing to prove. But he knows if his heart isn't in it, if he's feeling dejected himself, things might go wrong. There's a life on the line, and while John may be doing it tough, he'd never compromise on patient care.

When I get out of the ambulance just north of the lighthouse and head towards the cliff I hear John's door slam behind me and I know that he's following. We're partners and he's always got my back, no matter how bad he's feeling. I'm grateful for his loyalty.

We've beaten the cops to the scene and the talk-down falls to me. On the other side of the fence, on the lip of a rock jutting out above the sea, sits a man in his thirties. He wears little round glasses, like John Lennon did, and his shoes are on the ledge, neatly placed beside him. John hangs back as I make the approach.

I introduce myself, gently. I don't want to startle him and cause him to fall.

His name is Martin, and he explains that he was checking Facebook in the early afternoon when he stumbled on a picture of his ex-boyfriend Simon cuddling another man. Devastated, he jumped in his car and raced up here with every intention of ending his life.

'I could've made the relationship work,' he says, sniffing. 'I had a chance with him. I'll never find anyone like Simon again.'

I look over my shoulder and see John's out of earshot. Listening to a patient with a similar story to your own can be especially difficult.

I try fishing for something in the man's life that might make him change his mind.

'You have parents?' I ask him.

He nods. 'Yes, my mum.'

The mum is the key, almost always the key.

'She loves you very much, doesn't she?'

He thinks for a moment, then says, 'Yeah, she does.'

Occasionally this strategy doesn't work. Some people have less-than-harmonious relationships with their mothers. Or their depression is so severe that even the love for a mother can't save them. The risk of a talk-down going wrong is ever present. One false move and the patient is gone, but Martin's scared and he's sober. I'm feeling confident he won't go through with it.

It begins to rain lightly. There are raindrops on Martin's glasses; he takes them off and folds them up, puts them down beside his shoes. He moves closer to the edge and drops his legs over. His body is shaking with fear.

Nothing's for sure, and now, as he inches closer to losing his balance, my confidence fades. I start to think he will actually do it. Why else would he take off his shoes and his glasses? Why anyone would care about their glasses getting shattered on the rocks or lost in the water is beyond me. But taking them off is symbolic.

Police Rescue, who've been getting harnessed up behind me, make hand signals that indicate their readiness to act. I consider giving them the nod, as Martin is now in a delicate spot. If he sees them approaching, things could go badly. Rescue know how to win people over, but they can also see I've built a rapport so they leave me alone. Suicidal people are quickly exhausted by sharing their woes over and over with different negotiators. My priority is coaxing Martin from the edge and convincing him to put his glasses back on. I need to buy time before I bring in the others.

As if in answer to my thoughts, I see a humpback whale a hundred metres out to sea. It catches my eye as it launches from the ocean in majestic slow motion, a glorious sight. The whale seems to pause in midair, surrounded by spray, before dropping back gracefully into the swell. Never have I seen a migrating whale this close to the cliffs.

'Martin, look! The most beautiful whale, just out there. Put your glasses on, quick!'

He turns to the ocean, realises he can't see a thing, then fumbles for his specs and puts them back on.

'Where? Where is it?'

We look, but there's nothing. The whale's gone back under.

'I can't see it,' he says.

'Ah, whales. You know how they are. After jumping they go for a dive, and no matter how long you stand there and watch they might never come up. In saying that, we could always get lucky. You never know.'

Martin sighs and looks doubly depressed. I've made him feel worse: from a failure in love to a failure in whale watching.

'Believe me,' I tell him, trying to win back some ground that I've lost, 'that whale was a beauty. Isn't life worth it, to see that?'

But he wasn't a witness, and I feel like an idiot. At least his glasses are back on his face.

The rain falls steadily now and John comes up behind me carrying a blanket. He's probably impatient, and I worry at first that he's going to play bad cop.

'This is John,' I say. 'John, meet Martin.'

'Come on, guys,' says John. 'It's about to piss down. I've got a nice warm blanket. Martin, let's have a chat in the ambulance, out of the rain, okay?'

Martin nods. 'Can I call my ex-boyfriend?' he asks.

'Of course,' says John.

His kind and firm approach seems to have worked. It never takes him long to have patients eating out of his hand.

Martin climbs back over the fence and puts his arms around me. He cries into my shoulder before we start the slow walk to the ambulance.

After the job John says, 'Honestly, do you really have to hug them?'

He makes me laugh.

'It's *them* hugging *me*, okay?' I reply.

What I don't say is that John's just as guilty as I am with hugs. He too gives them out when the moment is right. Often it's all that a patient will need.

★

It's dark by the time we reverse into the plant room of the ambulance station. We've worked nearly thirteen hours straight and both of us are spent.

'It's depressing, all these depressed people, don't you think?' John says as he mops out the back of the ambulance. I recognise the feeling. I too have worked shifts in the shadow of the black dog while comforting others in similar states.

As he tips out the mop bucket he says, 'When I started in this game it was car crashes, heart attacks, drownings, *real* shit. Not people feeling sorry for themselves, crying and carrying on. Tell me, have you ever called an ambulance because you felt depressed?'

In my twenties I suffered a bout of depression, for less than twelve months. Relationship problems before I met Kaspia and too many overtime shifts were to blame. I guess a year is not long to be feeling depressed, but a doctor was worried enough to prescribe medication. After ten months I stopped it. Am I depressed now? I don't think so. I'm sad, and feel lonely at home, but I'm also optimistic. The breakup with Kaspia is temporary; we still have feelings for each other.

I say, 'Depression is a sickness. I had it once too.'

John looks up, surprised. Then he turns and puts the mop in the bucket. 'Sorry, didn't know. But still, tell me, did you ever call an ambulance for it?'

'No, I didn't.' Although it's fair to say that, like many paramedics, there isn't much I'd call an ambulance for. It runs in the family. I recall a story about my father's grandfather, who fell into the harbour from a Sydney ferry at Circular Quay on a rainy winter's day. He suffered a nasty laceration to his leg on the way down. Once he fished himself out with his umbrella and briefcase, the ferry master offered to call him an ambulance, but he refused. Instead, he bought a copy of the *Sydney Morning Herald* and laid it out on the back seat of a taxi, which he took to Sydney Hospital to have himself stitched up. My grandmother Murial was equally resilient, with a no-fuss attitude. She was hit by a bus in her eighties and got to her feet, brushed herself down and carried on walking. She wouldn't have been able to do that had she had a serious injury, of course. But it shows what we're made of.

'If you or I called an ambulance, we'd just be worried about who they'd send us. What if we got a pair of dickhead paramedics?' says John.

'Luckily there aren't many of those,' I reply.

But the real issue is our colleagues finding out about our breakdowns. There's a learned mindset in this line of work that vulnerability is a liability. It may be the same for other professionals, but for them privacy can be maintained when emotional cracks appear. I've treated politicians, CEOs and celebrities with mental health disorders and drug addictions, some of them after suicide attempts. They all know we're bound to keep their identities secret. We use separate radio channels or phone networks, we cover their faces or disguise them and organise private rooms at hospitals. Their employees or fans will never find out. But the same can't be said for paramedics. When paramedics pick up other paramedics, it doesn't take long for the whole service to know, as our colleague Hamish discovered. Your sanity and competence come into question, and your reputation and future feel threatened.

'If you're genuine, you'll go through with it,' John says. 'Serious players don't call. If they reach for the phone it means they're okay. Okay enough to speak to a shrink or Lifeline or a friend or whatever. Not paramedics. People don't call us because they *might* break a leg. But they call because they *might* kill themselves.'

'Because that's what we do, prevent people dying.'

'If they've made the decision to call, they've saved themselves already. Their inner voice has talked them down. No ambulance required.'

I change the subject. 'What does your inner voice think about a drink at the Bondi Hotel?'

'My inner voice says *Dancing with the Stars*.' It's his favourite show on TV.

As much as I want to help John, some lines I can't cross. Only after he backs out of the plant room and drives into the night do I think I could've made an exception and joined him for *Dancing with the Stars*. Maybe I'd even enjoy it. Could it be any worse than going home alone? But it's too late; he's already left.

CHAPTER 10

At dawn the next day there's not a cloud on the horizon over Bondi Beach and the sea is glassy, almost flat. Coming down the hill from the south, I can make out just a few infant waves lapping at the morning sand. Some desperate surfers might try to ride those later: tourists mainly, learners.

When I pull in to the station behind John's car I see Jerry in the plant room waiting for us. He's coming off a night shift, standing there moving back and forth on his feet like he needs to take a leak.

'Check this out,' he says with amusement, holding up a newspaper for John and me to see. It's the latest issue of *SX News*, the free gay and lesbian rag available across East Sydney. 'You're famous.'

On page three of the newspaper is an article on drug use in gay saunas, penned by the German manager of Ken's of Kensington. The man begins his tirade against the prevalence of amphetamines, amyl nitrate and GHB by recounting the story of the patient John and I revived on the transparent floor of his establishment two weeks earlier. And there, about halfway through the article, he writes of his gratitude that the ambulance service dispatched 'two brilliant gay boys' to his sauna.

John's face lights up with a grin, and my stunned expression sends Jerry into a fit of giggles. 'Two brilliant gay boys! Did you read it? Fantastic!' He slaps me on the back. 'How long you been a *brilliant gay boy* for, mate?' No doubt Jerry thinks he's got me. But it isn't the first time as a well-groomed, well-spoken man with theatrical flair that I've been mistaken for a homosexual. And it doesn't, and shouldn't, offend me in the slightest.

The article has certainly brought some morning fun to the station. Even John seems cheery.

As office workers head into town, crawling along in peak-hour traffic, we edge our way around them and against the oncoming cars, our siren wailing. A man in Glebe is having chest pains and all the Redfern ambulances are occupied. We're the closest available resource.

Turns out the patient, Edward, is a qualified hypnotherapist who says he was an ambo at Bondi back in the early 1970s. We treat him for a heart complaint and take him to Royal Prince Alfred Hospital, in the inner west suburb of Camperdown. On our way there he tells us how he went straight from military service in Vietnam to ambulance service in Sydney. Edward recalls that the rate of road trauma in an era of non-existent seatbelt and drink-driving laws was high and that, tortured by nightmares of Vietnam, he found it difficult to contend with the blood and guts of ambulance work. It was common at the time for officers to respond to calls on their own, and he went to shootings, fatal crashes and, like us, suicides at The Gap. Even the career of actress and singer Marlene Dietrich came to a halt in his ambulance one night when she hit the bottle a little too hard before her show and toppled off the Opera House stage. According to Edward, Dietrich badly fractured her hip, ending up at St Vincent's with an injury she never recovered from.

Back then the ambulance service was a conservative, military-style outfit; ambos wore ties and peaked caps and marched in parades. Edward's superiors took exception to his long hair and earrings and rainbow beads. After finding out about his daily marijuana habit they told him he was no longer fit for duty. Edward had already decided to resign, anyway. There were enough ghosts chasing him from his army days and he didn't need more.

Soon after leaving the ambulance service, Edward lost his apartment and began to live rough under the Andrew 'Boy' Charlton Pool near the Art Gallery of New South Wales. He stayed there for eighteen months, before a man who regularly swam at the pool saw him one day and picked him up by the collar. The man dragged Edward to hospital for help. The good Samaritan left his details, and when Edward cleaned himself up he contacted the man to offer his thanks. Before long the two of them fell in love.

'So you're still with this guy?' asks John.

'Been with him ever since. Never looked back.'

John grunts, and his grunt sounds cynical to me. If he wasn't in uniform he might've said, 'Enjoy it while it lasts.' Love is a dirty word for John right now. To him, no fairytale about a man transformed by love could possibly end well.

There's been many a short career in ambulance work. Some leave because of bad backs from carrying patients down stairs or dragging them out of crashed cars. Others, like Edward, have been rocked by post-traumatic stress. Nowadays paramedics are as likely to resign from the boredom and banality of the calls: the UTIs and common colds we're presented with, and the social work that makes up much of our day.

Outside a cubicle in the emergency department of Royal Prince Alfred Hospital, I bump into a guy I used to go to high school with. His name is Hugh, and his thick eyebrows and long face remain unchanged. He was the biggest and meanest bully in my year and I was one of his prime targets. He also thought I was gay, and no amount of protest convinced him otherwise. Like those nightclub bouncers who assault punters in CCTV blind spots, Hugh never missed a chance to hit me when the teachers weren't looking.

Seeing him in that hospital bed, I don't shrink in fear or turn on my heels as I once might have done. Seventeen years after graduation I'm far from the awkward, timid teenager I used to be. Within a year of joining the ambulance service I was out of my shell and presiding over life-and-death situations, bringing order to chaos with command and control. I had a uniform and respected skills. I'd never take bullshit from a bully again.

This time it's *Hugh* who shrinks from *me*. As I approach him he sees my uniform, and I can tell he's recognised me. His eyes widen in fright, as if anticipating a vicious revenge, but I just feel sorry for him. He looks so helpless in that cubicle, so vulnerable in his backless hospital gown. I approach him with a friendly smile.

'Hugh!' I shake his hand. 'What're you doing here?'

He looks around nervously, checking that no one has seen or heard us speak.

'Took an overdose,' he tells me in a hushed voice, almost a whisper.

'What of?'

'Antidepressants.'

'I'm sorry to hear that, mate,' I say.

'Listen,' Hugh says with a face creased in worry, 'don't tell anyone, okay? Please. I don't want anyone to know about this. Promise me?'

I reassure him that I don't keep in touch with many of the 'old boys', and I wouldn't tell them anyway. Hugh might once have ruled the playground, inflicting insults and violence on other kids, but even then, when he towered over me with his fists raised, surrounded by his accomplices, I could see right through him. He was chronically insecure, and when I look into his eyes now there's fear, just like the fear I once felt in his shadow.

Before leaving the hospital I say goodbye to Edward, and he gives me his contact details. You never know when a trusty hypnotherapist might come in handy, he tells me. Edward says he'll write the ambulance service a letter of appreciation about us. He knows thank-you letters are attached to our files, help keep us in the good books.

Back at the ambulance I tell John about running into Hugh, the ex-bully. John tells me he had a similar experience last year on a job in Kings Cross, when he found his former head prefect overdosed on heroin in a squat. Funny how things turn out, he says.

Uncannily, our controller dispatches us to Potts Point minutes later to treat an unconscious male, a suspected drug overdose. We arrive at a narrow lane, a dead end, with less than a foot of room on either side. I reverse the wagon down it in case we need a quick getaway if things turn bad. John knows what I'm doing and why. After our last fortnight of volatile patients and relatives we can't be too careful.

At the end of the alley a man in a dirty tracksuit is standing over a body. The scene is a textbook heroin overdose, with the patient hardly breathing and his pupils so small we call them 'pinned'. At least he isn't in cardiac arrest like the pie-eater's flatmate. John moves the guy on his side and runs some oxygen through a bag and mask. We give him Narcan and wait for him to wake. Used condoms, wet tissues, bloody syringes and vomit are scattered around us. This is our workplace.

'Quite the popular alleyway,' John comments.

No wonder the disgruntled residents of a townhouse backing onto this spot have spray-painted FUCK OFF, JUNKIES on their garden wall. Though it's hardly been a deterrent.

John's only halfway through one of his favourite hospital sandwiches when we're sent to the Housing Commission's most notorious high-rise blocks, on Belvoir Street, Surry Hills.

People call them 'suicide towers' given how many people plunge to their deaths from the balconies.

Our patient's name is Hope, an African immigrant on the sixteenth floor. She cries and touches a bruise round her left eye. There's a wound on her head and clumps of her plaited hair lie on the carpet. Her boyfriend has beaten her up again, she tells us. He made some threats too, about sending a mob to kill her family back in Sudan. Hope sobs loudly and then, with lightning speed, she jumps onto the kitchen bench, slides open the window and tries to throw herself out.

John's impressively quick. He lunges for Hope's leg and grabs her ankle as her weight shifts, just in time. John wrenches her back into the room and the two of them fall onto the floor in a heap.

'That's it, Hope, you're coming with us,' he snaps.

We drop her off at RPA and, when we return to the ambulance, I commend my partner for his reflexes.

'Ironic, isn't it,' he says. 'Her name. She'll be discharged and back there tomorrow, you wait.'

Or maybe not. People *do* get out of their suicidal thinking with intervention – some of them, at least, the ones without a serious mental illness. And even the latter can be helped. Suicide is preventable, people's lives can turn around. Problem is, as paramedics, we rarely see the follow-ups, the positive results, the transformations. We just talk them down and drop them off and go to the next one. When I make this point to

John he says, 'Revolving door, that's what it is. Revolves until they achieve their aim.'

'It doesn't revolve forever,' I say. 'People get better. Life's like that. Hills and valleys.'

John's annoyed. 'Hills and valleys? Some fucking valleys never become hills again. You thought about that? Some valleys go on and on, far as the eye can see. Desolate plane.'

A few hours later we head to St Vincent's with a patient suffering flu. She requested a lift because 'people on benefits can't afford taxis'. We don't argue. John could do with a dose of his fun-loving nurse mates in Emergency, anyway. The hospital is a social club for doctors, nurses and paramedics as much as it is a place for the sick and injured. Standing around our stretchers we gossip like hairdressers, occasionally forgetting our patients can hear every word.

'Nice earrings,' John compliments Suzy, the triage nurse.

John and Suzy are long-time friends. She gives him a hug, tells him not to worry about Antonio, things might still work out, they often do. John chokes up a bit so Suzy takes him by the arm and out into the ambulance bay for a heart-to-heart. She's good at those. These nurses owe him one. It's usually John who's counselling *them* about *their* love lives. Straight women seeking a gay man's advice on romance might be hard to understand, but many seem to want it. Only men can truly know the secrets of pleasing men, John once explained to me. And he's been pretty good at keeping a man too. Until now.

John and I pick up a forty-year-old woman with abdominal pain. Her name is Karen and we think she's got pancreatitis; we're not sure. Whatever the cause, she describes her pain as severe but flatly refuses our offer of morphine. I give her an alternative, methoxyflurane, and she happily inhales it until she's pain-free and rather high. Methoxyflurane is a central-nervous-system depressant better known to the public as the 'green whistle'. It has a few side effects, but those that aren't mentioned in the literature are loquaciousness, feelings of sexual desire and properties that have led us to call it a 'truth serum'. Once peak levels are reached, secrets of all kinds gush forth unhindered by fear or shame, often in the presence of people from whom these secrets have long been kept.

Karen's anxious husband is riding up the front with John when she drops the bomb.

From the back of the ambulance she calls out, 'Graeme? Graeme! Guess what? I know you've been having an affair with Alice. I've known for ages. You can't hide it anymore.'

There's a deathly silence.

Graeme turns around and I see his face has lost all colour. 'What? What did you say?'

Karen sucks on the green whistle again like she's puffing

on a Cuban cigar. 'I said, I know you've been fucking Alice. And, let me tell you, since I found out about that, I've been fucking Roger.'

'Roger?' Her husband sounds alarmed. '*Roger* Roger?'

'*Roger* Roger,' confirms Karen.

It's never been so awkward in our ambulance. Neither John nor I dare interrupt their conversation, although John briefly turns to glance at me with a look of amusement.

Before I'm able to stop her going on, Karen says to me, 'Don't get me wrong. I *do* love my husband. See him up front? See how sexy he is? See his sexy profile? You know what my special name for him is? Donkey Cock. That's what I call him, yes I do. Donkey Cock. And it's *so* true! I'm telling you, the thing is just *enormous*.'

Graeme cranes around to look at us again. He's been listening to everything. It's a nightmare for him, this ambulance ride, this red-and-white confessional on wheels. Distracted, John swerves to miss a car and slams his hand on the horn.

'Graeme? Can you hear me?' shouts Karen between tokes on the whistle. 'I know all about it, Graeme! You think I don't know, but I know. I know what you've been up to with Alice. But I only did it once with Roger, last year. Truth is, I love you, baby. It's *you* I love, Graeme! I *don't love* Roger at all. Can you hear me? Donkey Cock?'

Graeme is presumably too shocked to answer. Only the sound of our ambulance rattling over the bumpy lane on Oxford Street can be heard. John does the most sensible thing and switches on the stereo. He turns it up full volume. It's Elton John singing 'Tiny Dancer'. By the time we pull up at the hospital, Graeme looks like he needs a green whistle himself, while Karen is happily hollering the lyrics at the top of her lungs.

In the afternoon, the body of a woman is found washed up on a small nudist beach at Lady Bay. One might expect the naked sunbathers would pack up their summer picnics and go home at the sight of a white corpse lolling in the shallows. But the dead woman deters no one.

The cops reckon she's another 'gappie' – their term for a jumper from The Gap – and her body, now bloated, is tossed against the rocks by innocent waves. After falling off the cliff on the other side of the headland several days ago she must have been washed into the harbour.

'They're going over three a week,' says John to the cops.

'Bad year for it, eh. Bad year,' says a senior sergeant, wiping sweat from his brow.

December is ordinarily the busiest month for suicides. Some of us attribute this spike to lonely people having the communal festivities rubbed in their faces. Other experts blame the sunlight, a counterintuitive explanation given what we assume about seasonal moods: for me, winter is miserable and summer lifts my spirits. But despite Greenland having the highest suicide rates globally, statistics show that Northern Hemisphere suicides peak in June and Southern Hemisphere suicides in December. The theory is that increased hours of sunshine boost the energy and motivation required to go through with the act.

John and I watch from a low cliff above the beach as tanned men flex their muscles and parade their penises. Lying on a tartan blanket less than twenty metres from the dead body are two nude men clinking champagne glasses and laughing loudly. Further up, an old man slips into the water and begins an elegant breaststroke. None of them has noticed the floating cadaver at the end of the beach.

The Rose Bay police inspector appears through some bushes with a laminated map and clipboard, patting down his hair and waving a fly from his face. The inspector's phone rings and he walks off to have a conversation. Half a minute later the Police Rescue boys arrive wearing Santa hats. They rig up their abseiling gear and take off their utility belts, resting them on a boulder.

One of the rescue guys asks us to keep an eye on their guns. Then they abseil over the edge.

John looks at the weapons lying there, then across at me. I'm not quite sure what he's thinking, but judging by the mischievous twinkle in his eye he's probably imagining we could grab the guns and rob a bank. But the police inspector finishes his call and is already making his way back.

A geriatric birdwatcher, wearing a khaki safari suit drenched in sweat, stumbles out of the scrub. He apologises profusely, then asks if any of us has spotted a yellow-faced honeyeater in the area. We shake our heads and he disappears into the bushes again. Shortly afterwards we see a fully laden pleasure craft belonging to Captain Cook Cruises heading towards our escarpment, before suddenly veering away. The captain must have noticed the unpleasant view he was about to expose his Christmas party revellers to. Then, on the other side of the beach, we spy a press photographer clambering along a rock ledge nursing a giant telescopic lens.

'It's all happening here at Lady Bay,' says John.

The police inspector grunts. 'Guess I should speak to that guy,' he says of the photographer. The press usually avoids suicide stories, as some can encourage copycat trends. 'The paper won't publish a picture of this anyway,' says the inspector.

As we wait for the police helicopter, the inspector recounts his Gap stories. Several years ago, he says, a woman launched off the top but had second thoughts and grabbed a branch sticking out from the cliff face halfway down. She clung there until Police Rescue got to her and saved her life.

We leave the body for the police, who are making Lady Bay a crime scene. John and I head back to the ambulance through the shrubbery. Suddenly John stops and holds up a hand. 'Shhhh!' he says, pointing in the direction of a low bush.

There, sitting among the branches, is a small, yellow-cheeked bird we can only assume is the rare honeyeater the birdwatcher was searching for.

We look at each other in disbelief.

While fuelling up in the last hour of work we get our final emergency for the day: a woman feeling dizzy at Westfield Bondi Junction. She 'leant too far into a freezer at Woolworths while trying to reach potato gems', and is now sitting on a bench outside the supermarket. John manages to wheel the stretcher down and parks it beside her. I give her a once-over and, as I deflate the blood-pressure cuff, she says, 'I'm okay now. I'd rather die in Woolies than go to hospital.' While I dread shopping malls, I hate hospitals more, and I tell her I understand.

She declines further assistance and promises to see her own doctor. As soon as she's walked away, John elbows me and nods to a large placard outside a liquor store.

'Have a look,' he says. 'Twenty per cent off Pure Blonde.'

Without a second thought he steers our empty stretcher into the bottle shop. I remind him again that we're in uniform, but he doesn't care. 'Rules are for fools,' he loves to say. So he looks around to be sure no one's watching, then heaves two cartons of beer onto the stretcher and covers them with a blanket. At the cashier he lifts a corner of the blanket so the guy can scan the boxes, then pays for the booze and wheels it to the ambulance.

'What's your problem?' he asks me, detecting my anxiety. 'Wasn't I discreet enough?'

'Discretion was there,' I say. 'But we're not supposed to . . . I mean, just think about the headline. I'm always thinking about the headline.'

'Fuck the headline. Aussies would *cheer* at the headline.'

John slides the beer-laden stretcher into the ambulance and slams the back doors.

As I'm about to walk out of the station after the shift, I notice a package in my pigeonhole. It's a small parcel wrapped in brown paper. I open it and pull out a square blue box, like the ones precious jewellery comes in. I open it with a creak and see my National Medal for ten years' service lying on a bed of velvet. It's like the medal soldiers get, finally delivered to me after twelve years in the job; who knows why there's been a delay. The medal is a brushed-gold disc with a red-and-blue ribbon. Above it is a small, striped bar I can attach to my uniform. I don't take it out of the box.

Of course I'm pleased to have a recognition from my employer, recognition for the hundreds of days and nights spent rushing round the city and country towns I've worked in, helping those in need. I don't want to be ungrateful, but this is not the type of recognition that sustains me; what does is the appreciation I get from patients and their families. Even simple words of encouragement from a colleague or manager mean more to me than a medal.

In any case, I feel like a fraud. How can the career of a paramedic who genuinely believes he's never saved a life be worth this reward? Is the medal just for turning up and having a go?

'Everyone gets it,' says John when I show it to him. 'Don't start thinking you're special.'

I close the box with a snap and toss it into my bag. Once I get home I bury it at the bottom of my underwear drawer, in the same dark place I keep the word 'hero'.

CHAPTER 11

A few days pass and I don't see John. I phone him but my call goes to voicemail. A roster change has partnered John with Barry, a veteran paramedic who smokes like a chimney. I don't work with Barry much. I had a run-in with him once, when I first got to Bondi, a shouting match in the stairwell. It started with an argument after a comment I made on the lack of decor at the ambulance station. I said, 'This station needs more art.' And he said, 'It's a fucking workplace, not your home.' A week later I came in and found a three-by-four-foot painting on the wall, a hideous abstract artwork Barry had picked up from a charity shop which looked like an HSC kid's major work gone wrong. Everyone thought it was terribly funny. Jerry even stuck a title under the painting, called it *The Gilmour.* I now get on well with Barry, but he and the others still bring in ugly pieces of art to hang on the walls as an ongoing joke.

It's possible that our station officer, Frank, has put John with Barry because he thinks John needs someone senior to get him on track. As far as managers go, Frank's one of the best. He passionately advocates for all of us, especially in recent times for John. It pains Frank, I know, to give John letters from higher up the chain, putting him on notice for 'unacceptable' sick leave. If we clock up eight or more absences in a twelve-month period, we get a written 'please explain'. The last time I saw John get one of these he scrunched it up and threw it across the room, right into the recycling bin. It was a brilliant shot. Frank couldn't help smiling when John did that, even after he said, 'I've had it, I'm going off sick!' and left for the day.

Not long before Christmas I cross paths with John as he's leaving the station after work. His hair is a mess, his face covered in stubble. I can't think of a time I've seen him unshaven. There are few paramedics as presentable as John usually is, but he's let himself go. Barry tells me he's been buying bottles of a codeine cough suppressant and taking it home to drink between beers. All of us worry about him, but we're not sure what to do.

I'm about to ask John how things are going with Antonio,

but his expression tells me all. Without a smile he gives a curt hello and is back in his thoughts, far away, too far to reach. When he pulls out from the station he narrowly misses a delivery truck.

I'm now working with Matt, the paramedic intern who Jerry's been training. Matt lives somewhere near Cronulla. He moved down from the Northern Rivers region after joining the service two years back. Matt's twenty-three, intelligent, quick-witted and a keen learner, but thankfully takes himself less seriously than many new recruits. He's good for a laugh, and has a great future ahead of him.

It's Christmas Eve and a jogger at Bondi has phoned about seeing an unconscious woman lying on the beach. The lifeguards are also responding. We pull up on Queen Elizabeth Drive and Matt says, 'It might be that chick who likes getting on *Bondi Rescue*.'

Could be, I think. The woman Matt's referring to has borderline personality disorder, and frequently travels to Bondi from her Campbelltown home with the sole intention of appearing on the popular reality TV show *Bondi Rescue*, which follows the beach's lifeguards. The way she usually attempts her stunt is by flailing about in the water, pretending to drown, sparking a rescue effort. If she's not in the mood for getting wet, she'll feign a seizure near the shoreline.

Everyone knows her by name: the lifeguards, the paramedics, the police. And she still makes it onto *Bondi Rescue* because she gives the audience the entertainment they want. The TV show, in turn, gives *her* the attention *she* wants. It's a symbiotic relationship.

But our patient today is not the regular pseudo-drowner. We've never seen her before. She's in her early twenties and is on her back with her eyes firmly closed, breathing quietly. The lifeguards say she can't be woken. The patient doesn't answer when I call to her, but I'm not convinced she's unconscious; her breathing's too quiet, as if she's asleep. I run my fingers across her eyelashes, and they flicker.

'Hi, we're Matt and Ben, we're paramedics. What's your name? We're here to help. Can you open your eyes?'

But the woman isn't interested in waking up. Matt unzips our kit and passes me the Glucometer. I tell the girl I have to prick her finger and check her blood sugar. She doesn't respond so I just do it, and she still doesn't stir. Her glucose is fine. I take her pulse, do a blood pressure, check her temperature and pupil reaction, a few other things. All unremarkable.

'Listen,' I say, more sternly now, 'sorry to do this, but we need to know you can wake up and make sure there isn't something medically wrong with you. I'll have to inflict some painful stimuli by pinching you, understand? It might hurt, so now's the time to wake up of your own accord.'

She's lucky to get an invitation to stop faking it, if that's what she's doing. Plenty of medics launch right in with painful stimuli, although I did hear that our colleague Frank once tipped a jug of water over a patient's head at the Hakoah Club a few years back, which was rather unorthodox of him. Our patient doesn't accept the offer to wake voluntarily, so I take a bit of soft flesh behind her upper arm and pinch it between my finger and thumb. Then I twist it a little, watching her face for a grimace. This pinch can wake the dead, but our patient doesn't move. I look at Matt and raise an eyebrow. He shrugs. Then I pinch again, harder still. Half a dozen times I do it, confident one of my killer pinches will get a reaction. But she doesn't flinch.

'What a tolerance,' I say to Matt. 'Incredible.'

Just as I'm about to give up and ask Matt to bring down the stretcher, her eyes spring open like those of a doll in a horror movie. She's suddenly alert, and furious. She begins to scream at the top of her lungs: 'Fuck you, motherfucker! What the *fuck* is with you? How dare you pinch me like that, you fucking fucker!'

We back away now, Matt and I, from the bear we've woken. In a rage she lunges for me, but she stumbles in the sand and falls forward.

'Please,' I say, 'I was just trying to see if you were okay.' My hands are raised in defence as she gets up again and starts swinging her fists. Then she stops and points a finger at me.

'I was fucking okay until *you* came along and pinched the fuck out of my arm, you bastard!'

She turns to the crowd of morning beach joggers who have stopped to see the action and pulls up her sleeve, holding her elbow in the air for all to see, waving it back and forth.

'Look at my arm, people! Take a good look! That fucker there pinched the hell out of me. That para-fucking-medic!'

People step forward and squint to get a better view of the woman's pinched arm. From where I stand I can just make out a few red marks I've left behind, and I start to feel guilty. Trying to make amends, I say, 'I'm sorry for pinching you. But I needed to know if you were unconscious. How can we help you?'

'Fuck off!' she yells back. 'That's what you can do. I'm reporting this assault to the police right now. I'm having you *fucking* charged!'

Then she picks up her handbag, shakes the sand from it, and storms up to Campbell Parade.

'She's heading to the cop shop,' Matt says.

'I know she is,' I say.

'What're we gunna do?'

We return to the ambulance and I tell Matt to drive as fast as he can to the Bondi police station. I'm hoping we can get there before the woman does. But as we head down Gould Street we see her going through the front doors, so we park outside and discuss our options.

'Ya gotta call the supervisor,' says Matt.

I agree. I phone the ambulance supervisor and tell him the story, and he suggests we return to the ambulance station and ring the cops from there, explaining the situation.

When we get back I phone the police station and manage to get onto the sergeant at the front desk, who's still in the process of taking the woman's complaint. I know him. It's Stuart: nice guy.

'She's pretty unhappy with you,' he says in a low tone. 'Did you see the welts on her arm? Bloody hell, was that you?'

'Yeah,' I say. 'Didn't know she bruised that easily. I was just trying to wake her up. It's painful stimuli, it's what we do if a patient doesn't rouse to voice.'

'She's a bit psycho,' says Stuart. 'But you know, we have to investigate. Sorry, mate.'

'You going to charge me?'

Stuart laughs. 'Maybe. But don't lose any sleep, okay?'

Then he hangs up. Even though I know Stuart, even though he laughed, I'm not sure if he's serious or not. He has a job to do, after all. I start to feel nauseous.

'They gunna charge you?' asks Matt.

'Don't know.'

Matt shakes his head. 'How come *she's* the one pretending to be knocked out for whatever crazy reason and *you're* the one who ends up feeling bad about it?'

I suppose next time I'll have to be more gentle, or try another method. In some countries I've seen paramedics poke their patients in the eye with a finger to wake them up.

But that's not a helpful thought right now. Imagine if I'd done that to the girl on the beach? She'd have me for blinding.

While I contemplate the dreaded idea of seeing in the new year behind bars, we're sent to another suicide attempt. I tell Matt how John and I have lost count of such cases this month, how some shifts they were all we attended.

'Suicide magnets,' says Matt with a dark chuckle. 'That's what you are.'

Margo, an obese woman with schizoaffective disorder, is one of our regulars. She's sitting in her unit with the police. She tells us she went to throw herself off the tenth-floor balcony of her Housing Commission block but couldn't get her leg over the railing.

'I'm too fat,' she says, matter-of-factly.

The lady next door saw her struggling to climb the railing and called the cops, but she'd given up by the time they arrived.

She tells us her teddy bear is suicidal too, asks if he can come to hospital with her. It's a grubby old thing, all matted and grey, with just a hint around one ear that it used to be pink. I guess stuffed toys can also be victims of negative learned behaviours, victims of their environment. We take pity on the bear too and allow him to come along.

I've always had a soft spot for Margo. She's a troubled

child stuck in an adult's body. But it turns out she's not completely harmless. When I try to sit her down at the hospital she gives me a terrible fright by pulling out a six-inch kitchen knife from the back of her tracksuit pants.

'Sorry,' she says, handing me the blade. 'It's just not that comfortable sitting on this.'

What's not comfortable is the number of troubled people who carry knives around, even innocent-looking patients with teddy bears.

The streets are jammed with people doing their last-minute Christmas shopping. Shoppers in a frenzy can be dangerous, and injuries are occurring at regular intervals. We hear our controller send an ambulance to a woman who walked into a display at David Jones, while another has fallen down escalators at Westfield and a third has fainted in the perfume section at Myer. We could've been dispatched to any of these. But we're the suicide truck and I'm the suicide magnet, as Matt says, and that's what we're called to next.

In a backstreet of Surry Hills, not far from the terrace where John lived with Antonio up until a week ago, a man is sitting in his car covered in a strange white powder. When he sees us approach he winds down his window and calls out, 'Stay back! Keep back! Get away from me!'

'Why?' asks Matt.

'I'm killing myself,' he declares.

Turns out the man is a chemistry professor who has broken up with his online lover, and is now attempting an unconventional suicide.

'See this powder here?' he says, holding up handfuls of it. 'I'm not telling you what it is. But it'll kill me in forty-eight hours.'

This has to be the slowest suicide attempt ever made.

'Bet you it's only self-raising flour,' I say to Matt quietly.

'But ya never know,' he replies. 'Better call it in.'

As I give my report by radio I imagine the palaver that's about to unfold with the police and fire hazmat converging on the scene, the street blocked off, crowd gathering and news choppers circling. In late 2001 a mad scientist in the US sent anthrax spores by letter to media companies and congressional offices, killing a number of people. The whirl of media attention around these anthrax letters caused a whole lot of copycat white-powder incidents in other countries, though most turned out to be nothing more than flour posted by troublemakers getting in on the hype. All this resulted in a high level of cynicism about white-powder incidents among emergency-service workers like us.

Matt and I sit and wait and watch as the fire brigade's hazmat team arrive, donning their bulbous spacesuits and setting up a shower tent. They drag the professor out of his car for a naked hose-down by the roadside so we can put him in our ambulance. The whole operation takes a good two hours. After a chemical analysis, the fire hazmat commander formally concludes that the white powder was indeed self-raising flour, no anthrax bacteria detected. Seems our patient wanted nothing more than to make a scene, which he did.

Time for one more suicide before the day is done, I say to Matt as we hit 6 pm. He laughs, but I don't. When we make ourselves available I'm relieved the final call is to a 'concern for welfare'. An old man in a high-rise Waterloo apartment block hasn't been seen for a while. It's an easy job. We'll break in with the cops and find no one home, and that'll be it.

The Housing Commission tower casts a long shadow across the terraces below. It's not the first time I've been to this particular block. Last year a woman fell from the top and landed on the concrete below. Her curtain flapped like a flag in the breeze through her open window. I covered her body with a blanket and the blood soaked right through.

Today, a group of residents on the fifth floor are worried about the old man in 5534. Most days he leaves his place to buy bread, milk and a packet of cigarettes at the corner store. He usually does this around midday, says the woman in the apartment next door. But for the past week she hasn't seen him, and he won't open up when she knocks. He's in his eighties, she tells us; he might've tripped over.

'I've got his key,' she says. 'But he's got something jammed against the door.'

Matt calls for a rescue truck. As we wait in the corridor Matt says, 'I saw a poster with your missus on it. She still doing shows?'

'Got one coming up, after New Year's,' I reply.

'You helping her out?'

'We're taking a break.'

'Yeah, I know. You okay?'

'Sure. It's only short term.'

'John's taking it hard with Antonio, I hear.'

'Yeah, he is.'

Police Rescue arrive, carrying tools. They get to work and jimmy the door, but can't get it open more than a foot. One of the rescue guys makes a wedge with his boot and looks over at me.

'Just enough room for an ambo your size,' says the cop.

He must be joking. I turn to Matt and say, 'Junior officers first, right?'

'They don't call you Snake Hips for nothing!' Matt says with a laugh.

Bastard. The rescue guy chuckles. 'Snake Hips, eh? Well come on then, in ya go.'

Fussing about any longer would frustrate me more than the dirty work. When I crouch down it's easy to see there's no way my whole body will make it through the door, so I squeeze my head in for a little look around. Once my eyes adjust to the gloom, it appears the place is empty. But then, as I twist my head to the right, I see the legs of a man behind the door. My heart skips a beat. Has the sneaky bugger been quietly standing there while we've all been knocking? Why would he play such a game? Then I notice his feet aren't touching the ground.

I pull my head back into the hall.

'One for you, gentlemen,' I say to the cops. 'He's hanging behind the door.'

As we leave the building I contemplate the lives that have ended here. The building is a repository of worn-out men and women with deeply tragic stories: lives spoiled by drugs and alcohol, marriage breakups and mental illness. I was at the same building with John just last month, when he told me he'd rather kill himself than end up living in a dark, mouldy room as small as a jail cell.

Before I leave work I call John's number. Again it goes to voicemail. I leave him a message, wishing him 'as happy a Christmas as can be expected', ending with the offer of a Christmas cake delivery. There's also a hamper of condiments, figs, chocolate and European biscuits that the producers of *Bondi Rescue* have sent the ambulance station. I could always drop some to John in the morning.

*

I spend Christmas Eve at my parents' house. Our family Christmas celebrations follow my German mother's tradition of *Weihnachten.* We help prepare a feast, light candles and sing carols. Before gifts are exchanged my father reads the story of the birth of Jesus from a leather-bound Bible, and says a prayer for the year ahead. My parents tell tales from our youth, and my brothers and sister and their partners laugh and clink their wine glasses. It's all very merry.

I try to act jovial, but I'm not convincing anyone. It's the first Christmas I can remember that Kaspia and I haven't been together, and it hurts. I've been stoic until tonight. I feel Kaspia's absence in every moment, and it's an absence that no one wants to talk about. In spirit I'm not present, either. I understand, just a little, how Christmas for some can exacerbate loneliness, depression and intrusive thoughts of suicide.

The streets are always quiet on Christmas morning. People's relentless rushing has finally been stilled. Scores have left on their holidays up or down the coast, others are overseas and the rest are at home with their families. But the paramedic roster, like the wheel of life, keeps rotating.

Matt and I spend Christmas Day driving past barbecues and laughter on the beach and parks of Bondi. It would have been harder spending Christmas Day without Kaspia if I wasn't on this shift. At least I can tell myself we're apart because of work, and not for any other reason. But I still check my phone far too often to see if she's sent a message or if I might've missed a call.

By midday, we haven't had a job yet.

'Let's not get complacent,' says Matt. 'There's always a handful of tragedies on Christmas. One of them might be ours.'

A couple of hours later one of them is.

After picking up a few jolly drunks, including an Irishman dressed up as Santa, we're called to a grandfather who has collapsed on his patio. His wife is crouched beside him, crying, 'Please help him, he's not breathing.' The rest of the family are huddled nearby, including his grandchildren.

Matt unbuttons the man's shirt and I stick on the defib pads. The rhythm's a flatline and no one's done CPR. We work on him for twenty minutes, but get no result.

I tell the man's wife that we're sorry, that there's nothing more we can do. Her husband of fifty years has passed away.

She takes his head in her hands and strokes his hair, telling him, 'Thank you, Henry, darling Henry. Thank you for being such a wonderful husband.' Then she cries out, 'I'm in a dream, a bad dream, a nightmare . . .'

I've heard this before, many times, the bad dream that people long to wake up from, the disbelief. I'll surely feel this one day too, but for now I can only imagine what it's like.

I get up and go to the mantelpiece, keeping my composure. I look at the couple's whimsical pet rock collection. Their neat row of Christmas cards. Photos of their grandchildren remind me they're in the house too, being shielded from this. The violence of chest compressions, needles in veins and tubes in throats wasn't for them. I take a deep breath and go give them the news. They read my face before I speak, but I say my piece anyway. 'We tried our best but he didn't pull through.' It's a worn phrase that makes it sound like it's the old man's fault, as if he refused to come back. 'We tried our best' sounds inadequate too. It may be true that we tried our best, but I wonder if *trying* is good enough. In our line of work, where the opposite of success is death, there's no prize for trying.

I wonder if love's like this too, if this sense of failure and recrimination follows you around when the pulse of a relationship stops. All those years of investment, the sweat and the tears, the battles to save it, for what? If my relationship with Kaspia ends, or if John and Antonio's does, will there be any comfort in saying, 'We tried'?

CHAPTER 12

It's the day before New Year's Eve, and an Air Ambulance plane from Broken Hill is due to come in to Mascot with a patient for St Vinnies. I'm back on with Jerry and he volunteers to drive. On the way out to the airport he tells me about Christmas with his wife and his kids and I tell him about Christmas with the grandchildren of a dead man.

'You didn't wish them Merry Christmas as you left, did you?' Jerry asks.

'What do you take me for?'

'We all say dumb things, mate.'

'No, I *didn't* wish them Merry Christmas as I left.'

We slip into a window booth at Krispy Kreme, opposite the Air Ambulance base. There's a good view of the hangar from here so we can see when the plane arrives. Jerry orders two cappuccinos and a small plate of cinnamon donuts. I sip on my coffee and ask him if he's been in touch with John. 'I tried calling Christmas Day, but he didn't pick up,' I say. 'From what I've heard he's been having more sickies. He looked like a tramp when I saw him last week.'

'Maybe we should search for him in Woolloomooloo,' Jerry says with a mouthful of donut.

'Funny you say that. He talked about moving down there if he had to. Joking, of course.'

'Or *not* joking,' says Jerry. 'I spoke to him before Christmas, you know.'

'So he answered your call?' I turn to Jerry.

'Yeah, but don't get offended he didn't answer yours. He's hardly talking to anyone. Maybe just his parents and sisters up the coast. A couple of friends. He only picked up because I redialled his number for an hour and it pissed him off.'

'Is he getting any help?'

'A shrink, so he reckons. Who knows.'

Our conversation is interrupted by a kid about twelve years old, who approaches from the next booth, where his parents are sitting. He sidles right up, says he loves paramedics.

'Thanks, matey,' replies Jerry. 'Very nice of you.'

The boy smiles, then pulls out a glossy Baptist Church pamphlet and lays it on the table. *How to avoid Hell!* is printed on the front. He slides it over to Jerry.

Jerry picks up the pamphlet and inspects it earnestly. The kid sits next to him, watching Jerry's face, waiting for questions or, even better, a sudden conversion. Jerry takes another donut and starts eating as he reads, then he looks up at the boy.

'Son, do you know what a *whoremonger* is?'

The kid is stumped. He shrugs.

Jerry goes on, 'Says here that a *whoremonger* is an example of the type of person who'll be going to Hell. This is very harsh stuff you've got here, you know? You really need to fully understand what you're handing out. It's only fair. Now, go back to your parents please, and ask them very nicely what a whoremonger is, okay?'

The boy, who doesn't quite know what to make of Jerry, takes the leaflet and retreats to the safety of his family.

'It's not that I don't want to *avoid* Hell,' Jerry says to me. 'But I don't think it's for humans to tell other humans who'll be going there.'

I couldn't agree more.

Out the window I catch sight of the Air Ambulance plane approaching. We get up and brush the cinnamon from our uniforms, nodding politely to the Baptist family on the way out. Then we head over the road to collect our patient.

Alfred, the man we load up, has unstable angina and some dubious dysrhythmias we see on our monitor. He could slip into cardiac arrest any minute, so I put on our beacons for the ride into town and switch on the radio for a tune. AC/DC's

'Highway to Hell' comes on and I quickly turn down the volume, embarrassed. But Jerry won't have it. He shouts from the back of the ambulance, 'Come on! I *love* that tune. Turn it up, will you? There are no whoremongers in *this* ambulance. We've got nothing to worry about, do we Alfred?'

In a Randwick house of black leather lounges and glass table-tops, a forty-nine-year-old man is suffering food poisoning. Jerry picks up the bucket containing the man's vomit. Brow furrowed, he studies the contents as thoughtfully as he did the Baptist boy's brochure.

'Hmmm,' he ponders. 'You've been eating beetroot, haven't you? A dish with beetroot in it? Am I right?'

Curled up in the foetal position on his lounge, the man groans in the affirmative. Jerry swishes the bucket around, panning for more clues.

'Aha, I've got it. Cabbage! There's some cabbage here too, isn't there? I'm getting a good picture now. Let me guess. A steak? You had a steak, didn't you? With some cabbage and beetroot on the side?'

Clutching his stomach, the man nods.

'Excellent!' says Jerry, looking proud of himself.

We give the guy a drip, then leave him with some advice and a booking with the after-hours doctor service. Back in the ambulance Jerry says to me, 'The guy's forty-nine and calls an ambulance for gastro. Thousands of people vomit in this city every night. Imagine if all of them called.'

But everyday illnesses we think don't warrant an ambulance can be utterly catastrophic in the minds of sufferers. Paramedics are among the most resilient members of society helping many of the least resilient. On one hand it's a perfect match, the way it should be. On the other, our frustration at some of our patients is a constant challenge to suppress in public, though frequently expressed in private.

'You know what the guy needed?' says Jerry.

'What?'

'A can of Harden-the-Fuck-Up.'

'It comes in a can?'

'Yes it does, like a drink. Harden-the-Fuck-Up printed on the side in big gold letters.'

I feel like Harden-the-Fuck-Up has been part of the paramedic's private vernacular long before Mark 'Chopper' Read made it famous last year.

The radio's turned down but I'm pretty sure I hear our callsign being repeated at low volume.

'Job,' I say, nodding to the handset.

Jerry picks it up and replies.

We're assigned to a man with a stomach-ache in Maroubra, another patient vomiting.

Jerry and I sigh at the same time.

At least it's not a suicide.

★

A seventy-three-year-old man with a giant belly lies on his bed, his wife hovering anxiously nearby. She says her husband threw up after a sudden onset of abdominal pain. Our patient is very pale, sweaty and short of breath. It's no ordinary gastro, this one.

Unzipping the oxygen kit, I see the gauge level is nearly on zero and I curse quietly.

'You checked this earlier?' I ask Jerry.

'Yeah, what's up?'

'Almost out.'

I look closer. The regulator's come loose. Oxygen's been leaking all morning.

'Gotta get another cylinder,' I say. 'Sorry.'

Jerry shrugs and starts taking the man's blood pressure. But it's easy to see how low it is just by looking at him, so I call for backup on my way out the door.

I fetch another cylinder. When I come back I see Jerry on the bed straddling our patient and doing CPR. The two of them are bouncing up and down in the most ridiculous fashion. Jerry turns to me all puffed and says, 'Can't get him on the floor, too heavy. Give me a hand!'

We drag the man off the bed and onto the carpet. His head hits the rug with a thud. He's been incontinent and faeces is spread all over the place. I tear off his pyjama top and apply the defibrillator pads while Jerry continues chest compressions, trying to avoid the free-flowing shit.

The Lifepak 15 shows a bizarre and pulseless rhythm, one we can't shock. But Jerry, a former swimming champion, has muscular forearms and his compressions are excellent. They're so effective, in fact, that CPR is enough to give our patient a cardiac output and he starts to wake up. This only lasts half a minute, before he drops unconscious and loses his pulse again. Jerry jumps back on his chest. The man regains a pulse and wakes a second time, attempting to push Jerry's hands off his sternum.

These short periods of wakefulness are transient, seemingly generated by CPR alone. They are, most likely, the man's last lucid moments before his heart gives out permanently.

His wife stands with a hand over her mouth in shock. When the old man wakes again and looks around in bewilderment I tell him, 'Your heart keeps stopping and may stop for good. If you have anything important to say to your wife, now's the time.'

If I were the patient and a medic was telling me I had seconds to live, I'd like to think I'd find something meaningful to express to my partner, at least tell her that I loved her. But our man just stares at us, then at his wife, then back at us. I see on the monitor that his rhythm is starting to change, and I know he's about to slip away.

'Well?' I prompt him. 'Anything to say to your wife?'

But his stare becomes a glare, and all he says is, 'Nup.'

Then he flatlines and dies.

Later I feel bad for setting him up. Maybe there was too much to say in just a few seconds. Maybe he'd already told his wife how much he loved her and didn't want some paramedic directing the scene. Maybe their love language wasn't poetry, wasn't even verbal. Or maybe death is simply a private experience, as many believe it is, one that excludes all others, even life partners: a final pause of inward reflection.

In the wake of the man's death, Jerry and I sit down for a debrief over chicken curry at an Indian restaurant. Dipping a bit of poppadum in mango chutney, Jerry questions the point of some of our resuscitation attempts.

'Death's natural in old people, right? And the younger ones I've saved I reckon went back to their TV dinners, mouthing off and being the same slobs they were before.'

Either that, or they wind up brain-dead in nursing homes, which is what happened to the first two saves of a paramedic friend of mine from St Ives. The disillusionment about those cases nearly broke him.

'People in cardiac arrest I've treated seem to never leave hospital,' I say. 'They stay in ICU for a week until the family switch off life support.'

'You got the lucky streak, eh?' Jerry chuckles. 'Remind me not to take you to the races.'

My only consolations have been the hope that these

brain-dead patients are registered for organ donation, that their deaths may in some way help others have a better or longer life, and that families get a chance to say goodbye.

We pull away from the Indian restaurant and I tell Jerry about my brother Mark, how he saved a guy in the surf. Jerry says he also had a save not long ago, a famous actor in cardiac arrest on the beach.

'Far as I know, he's alive and well.'

It could've been me sent to that job, if I'd been on shift that day. It's strange, this feeling of jealousy again, the same I had with my brother's save. It's mostly luck of the draw: right place, right time. Even so, Jerry agrees that my saving of a life is long overdue.

'It's probably only my second one ever,' he says, trying to make me feel better.

'What was the other?'

'Ten years ago in the Cross. Guy was stabbed in the heart. Frank and I were parked around the corner having burgers. We got there in seconds. Just threw him on the stretcher, and I jumped on top like I did on that last bloke and I stuck my finger right in his heart while Frank floored it to St Vinnies. Guy pulled through.'

It's a remarkable story, especially as Jerry's pretty relaxed when it comes to the clinical stuff. Some think he's a slacker, but he just keeps his gunpowder dry. I've seen him work wonders on critical patients.

Jerry shakes his head. 'A good save for sure, but the guy was a scumbag. Big drug dealer, it turned out. Probably flogging bad shit to young kids a week later, messing up teenagers' lives, getting them hooked, killing them. When I think of that it makes me wonder if I really did the right thing, you know, sticking my finger in his heart.'

In a Waterloo park we know too well, there's a man lying in a bush. He's overdosed on heroin and we jab him with Narcan. A few minutes later he's awake. Instead of stumbling off, he looks at us and begins to cry.

'What's going on, buddy?' Jerry says.

'I always wanted to be a paramedic like you,' he sniffs, wiping his nose. 'It was my dream.'

'What happened?' I ask, putting a hand on his shoulder.

'Shit happened, that's what,' he replies, looking down at his track marks. 'I fucked up.'

We feel sorry for the guy. Fucking up is easy. I offer to find him a sandwich and orange juice at the hospital, get him some help, a referral to rehab perhaps. But he asks for a lift to Kings Cross instead, no doubt to score again. We take him to the hospital a few blocks from the Cross and watch him exit and walk down the road. I reflect on the part we have played in the cycle of addiction.

As we leave the hospital, Jerry mentions the name of a former paramedic we sometimes see shooting up at the injecting room on Kellett Street. Hers is another tragic story: a highly qualified woman who used to save victims of heroin in the nineties, when overdose deaths were rife. They say she burnt out and started taking morphine from the ambulance safe. After she got sacked she moved on to heroin. Every now and then we come across her doing mouth-to-mouth on an overdose victim before giving us a perfect handover laced with expletives.

Family conflicts are common this time of year, and we're frequently called to anger-related trauma. In a fit of rage a man has punched a window with such force that one of his fingers has been sliced clean off. He's out on the street and gripping his wrist in pain, his hand bound with a shirt. His amputated finger lies among shattered glass.

We wrap his finger in plastic and fold an icepack around it. Some people put their amputated parts directly on ice, but that can turn out badly. Once I treated a man who lost his nose after walking through a window and his friends put his snout directly on ice. When I went to fish it out it was stuck to an ice cube. Only after warming it with my breath was I able to peel the thing off.

As we drive to Sydney Hospital, Jerry says, 'Did you hear about the job the Naremburn ambos did last Saturday?'

'No. What?'

'They were kicking back at the station, watching a cooking show on the ABC, and the TV chef was slicing a carrot in a close-up and suddenly the screen cut to black and some unrelated promo comes on. Well, guess what? A minute later they're sent to ABC Studios for a lacerated finger.'

Even our patient, with one finger less, laughs out loud.

Christmas is over, but calls to The Gap haven't yet abated. Before 6 pm we're sent to Watsons Bay. We're relieved to see the cops already there, chatting to a woman who is standing like a statue on the edge, her black dress rippling in the breeze. Her name is Courtney. A young constable is doing the talking, but he's getting nowhere. 'Excuse me, miss!' he repeats, trying to get her attention, like a kid in a classroom. I offer to help.

'Go for it, mate,' he says with relief.

It turns out he wasn't loud enough. When I call to her she replies, 'I can't hear you!' It's the sound of the ocean, a big swell below, that drowns out our voices. I ask Courtney to take a step back so we can have a conversation. She turns and moves towards me, but only to take off her jewellery and lay it on the ground, before saying, 'Can you give this to Andrew?'

Andrew's my way in to the conversation. I ask about him and Courtney tells me how he's left her, how they're having a separation, and she's the one at fault. It sounds like she's had an affair that her husband's found out about. I tell her I'm separated too, that I'm hanging on to hope that things'll work out. But Courtney is talking with despair, talking more like John.

The constable comes over and whispers to me that Andrew's arrived at the scene. I ask the constable to wait with Courtney while I talk to the husband, who is standing with Jerry and the other cops about twenty metres away. Andrew is shaking, his eyes tense with fear. 'Tell her I love her. Tell her that, will you? I love and forgive her.'

When I go back to Courtney and pass on the message, she cries and says she doesn't believe me. She moves closer to the edge. The constable beside me says, 'She's gunna go, she's gunna go . . .' I ignore him and get Courtney's attention again. I tell her how genuine Andrew sounded about forgiveness, how fearful he looked.

'Think about the good times you could have with him again,' I say. 'He sounds like he adores you. Come on, take my hand, take it for Andrew, for yourself, for love.' She turns and steps towards me and takes my hand. The constable and I help her climb back over the fence.

As I carry Courtney's high heels to the ambulance I try to lighten the mood.

'How did I go?' I ask her.

She laughs through tears and says, 'Not bad, but a little bit Oprah.'

A little bit Oprah? John will love that when I tell him.

CHAPTER 13

New Year's Eve is a failure. I choose not to work it, hoping I'll be invited to a party, make some new friends. But my phone doesn't ring and I find myself walking down to Circular Quay on my own, through jubilant masses of couples and families, past smiling revellers with streamers and whistles and glow-sticks. I look for a place to watch the fireworks from, but I've left it too late. I get caught in a crowd crush on the corner of Albert and Phillip, behind the concrete monstrosity of the Cahill Expressway, which blocks out completely any view of the harbour. All I can do is listen to the fireworks, the whistling and cracking of rockets exploding, the thudding like that of incoming mortars, shaking the buildings and echoing through the city.

I've never cared much for new year's resolutions, and I'm

not superstitious. But Kaspia sees signs and omens everywhere, and I begin to worry that she might make some grand realisations and resolutions that will affect our future together, as she enters the new year alone.

I try going for a drink at a local small bar, but the other booths ring out with laughter and conversation as I sit on my own, looking like I expect company that never turns up. So I go home and lock myself away again. I write a little, and read and listen to some blues on vinyl. I don't need to go out; I have enough supplies. Over the course of four days I eat two-minute noodles, a handful of frankfurters, and a few meals I get delivered. I drink six beers. This would be several less than Jerry would've had, and considerably less than John.

As for John, late on my last day off I call his phone but it goes straight to voicemail. I think about getting out and driving down to see him uninvited, but change my mind. Then I consider going to Balmain for some lunch, hoping to bump into Kaspia, but change my mind about that too. No one likes a stalker.

My shift back with Jerry begins with the unexplained death of a man in his fifties. His apartment's another museum of loneliness: bottles of spirits, a marijuana bong, the director's cut of the French film *Betty Blue* on VHS. As far as we can tell there's no evidence of foul play, no self-inflicted wounds, no empty pill packets. Just a body, and the stagnant odour of isolation.

Guarding the scene when we leave is Wendy, the 'hottest cop at Waverley' according to her colleagues. She recently did a long-term undercover operation disguised as a sex worker in the Cross. She loitered on street corners with a lipstick and pistol in her handbag. When I ask her why she's back in uniform, she looks annoyed. Going undercover was the worst job of her career, she tells me. Not because of the criminals and customers, but because of all the pesky police cars doing laps of the block just to check her out in her miniskirt and knee-high boots.

Observing the talent on the street has always been a way emergency workers pass time between calls. Few of us can deny we've given running commentary on pedestrians – their fashions, their faces, their interactions – all from the safety of our ambulances. Only occasionally does a foolish paramedic overstep the line and wind down the window. Less than a month ago, Kaspia told me she'd been sitting at a bus stop on Oxford Street minding her own business when an ambulance crawled past and a paramedic leant from the passenger window and said, 'Hmmm, yes please!' Kaspia told me not to worry; she reminded me she was a burlesque dancer, and that it wasn't the first time she'd received such a comment. But for a good day or two I was furious.

★

A call to a George Street hotel forces us to scoff the dinner we've been eating in the front seat of the ambulance. In the foyer, one of the guests is hyperventilating. His chest is heaving, his hands are in a spasm.

The easiest treatment for anxiety-related hyperventilation is a paper bag over the face, or an oxygen mask on low. But there's a better way, a more challenging but sustainable solution to calm a patient down: reassurance and breathing techniques. Luckily, Jerry and I share a preference for the latter approach. We both enjoy the fun of running impromptu meditation sessions with our patients. As a qualified yogi, Jerry has quite the knack for it. So does John, when he's in the mood. And it's become a sort of challenge between the three of us: how quickly, without the aid of a paper bag, we can calm a patient down and bring their breathing back to normal.

Jerry sinks into a leather lounge near our patient and closes his eyes. He's telling me, in his own way, that he wants me to run the session today. I don't mind.

Pacing back and forth, I guide the patient through a meditation with creative visualisation. In his mind I paint the picture of a placid lagoon on a distant Pacific island. I take him drifting on the surface of these tranquil waters, gently, effortlessly, in the late afternoon. The foyer is quiet now, apart from my voice, which I try to make as lilting as a tropical breeze. The only sound my patient can hear is the distant hush of surf on the reef. I tell the anxious man that he's weightless, in body and mind. He lives here, in this perfect paradise, like a castaway. There are no worries in this carefree place.

Ten minutes in, the man is completely relaxed. His eyes stay closed when I'm done. And when I turn around it seems the rest of the guests in the foyer are in the same state. They all look asleep. I wake Jerry with a nudge and we quietly slip from the scene.

After lunch we get sent to a brothel we've been to before. It's been repainted in primary colours, though I can still see stains under the new coat as we carry our gear up the stairs. We pass rooms with nothing in them but a mattress on the floor and a scattering of used condoms and syringes. Reception's behind chicken wire, and the only room service the place offers is a courtesy ambulance call.

Before the injecting centre opened round the corner there were shifts where we'd get several overdoses at this place alone. Recently we revived a man in Room 18; he was unconscious, with a half-full syringe still hanging out of his arm. Before we could put the needle in a sharps container, a working girl who was hovering over us reached down and pulled it out of his vein, injecting herself with the leftovers.

Craig, an excitable Paddington paramedic with a closely shaved scalp glinting like chrome, arrives to help us with a combative drug-affected patient. But he only makes things worse. Craig crashes into the room as if entering a boxing ring. Rude or aggressive attitudes rarely succeed in the clubs and brothels of the Cross. Amphetamines and certain drug combinations can make people volatile, especially when they're extremely sleep deprived. These patients are as fragile as pick-up sticks but can blow up like landmines. To avoid being a trigger I always make sure I approach them cautiously, with a passive manner and disarming smile. It's not fail-safe, but I've found this demeanour reduces the chance of aggression.

Craig yells at a scarred man who's holding a cigarette between his teeth. 'Put that bloody smoke out, mate! We're using oxygen, for fuck's sake.' The whole room is full of drug-affected people who've come in trying to help, their eyes darting this way and that. When Craig barks orders they all begin to bristle. The smoking man gets up and tries putting his cigarette out on Craig's arm. Craig pushes him into another guy with jail tattoos, who promptly decks the smoking man, sending him flying onto the bed. In no time it's an all-out brawl, with the one and only exit blocked. Jerry asks for urgent police assistance on his radio. Into the mayhem of the fighting mob our patient decides to projectile-vomit. I've seen it coming and I press my body into a corner, using our oxygen bag as a shield.

Trapped by the brawl in another corner, Jerry calls out to me, 'Can you believe this time last week I was fishing?'

If only our partners, our friends, our children could see us in these moments, it might inspire greater patience when we come home cranky. The pressures of the job have certainly been a factor in the arguments I've had with Kaspia, mainly after night shifts. I'm forever asking her to judge my behaviour with consideration for the night I've had. But as much as our partners might try to understand, they never get to witness the wrestles in brothels, the screaming parents of critical children, or the times we lock eyes with the dying. They might attempt empathy, and for that we are grateful, but even a good imagination can't replicate the madness of reality.

As we circle Kings Cross, waiting for a call, it feels like we're cruising for business. In that sense we're not so different from the street-corner sex workers and dealers and pimps. We all make a living off the lost and the lonely, and not many people know these streets like we do, or work quite as late.

Like John, Jerry doesn't mind a chat with the working girls in the Cross. We park on Bourke Street off Darlinghurst Road, and the transgender girls fix their make-up in our side mirrors. John knows a few by name, as does Jerry.

'Did John tell you about the tranny who stole his defibrillator from the scene of an overdose?' says Jerry.

I shake my head.

'She was spotted a few hours later strutting along Victoria Street with it slung over her shoulder like a handbag.'

We laugh, and Jerry winds down his window and asks the women how business is going. They reply with baritone grumbles that it's slow, far too slow. I sense we're cramping their style, scaring off customers, so I start the engine and pull onto William Street.

Ten minutes later, as we cross the Forbes and Liverpool intersection, Jerry recognises one of the women who plies her trade outside the Christian Science Church. Her name's Belinda. When she sees Jerry she waves at us and smiles. I toot the horn for him.

'She's so lovely, a really lovely person,' he says. 'Last time we picked her up she asked me to be her boyfriend. Then she saw my wedding ring. Man, was she crushed.'

'I'm not so sure about that,' I say. I was there, after all. She was probably wondering why he had such a cheap-looking wedding ring. He'd bought it on eBay for a dollar, not wanting to wear his real one at work.

I tell Jerry I bumped into Belinda a few weeks ago, on a day off, at the Surry Hills post office. I was sending a Christmas package to some friends overseas when I caught sight of her at the island bench. She was holding a card with a laughing Santa on it, and it seemed like she was trying to think of something to write. She was thoughtfully turning a ballpoint pen between her finger and thumb. I watched her as I put my package together. She didn't recognise me, at least not at first, probably as I wasn't in uniform. After a while she gave up and just slipped the blank card into the envelope, then carefully wrote 'To Dad' on the front.

That's when I decided to speak up.

'Belinda? Hi, I'm the paramedic working with Jerry. We've picked you up a couple of times in the ambulance.'

'Oh, yeah!' She smiled and appeared a little shy, perhaps embarrassed she'd been identified by someone knowing a bit too much about her line of work.

'How's Jerry?' she asked. 'He's such a sweet guy; it's been at least a month since you guys took me in.'

'He's fine, always looking out for you near the church.'

'Yeah, a lot of people do,' she said, giggling.

When I asked about the card she sighed despondently. Her greatest wish was to spend Christmas with her father, she explained, but it wasn't going to happen.

'Last time he told me to only come home when I'm clean. I love him and I know he loves me, but I can't shake the addiction. Everything I do is for heroin.'

She said she was sending the card so her father would know she was still alive. I offered to help her write a few lines in it, but she said she had nothing to say, no positive update to give him. Then she spoke of the countless times she'd come close to getting off the street, away from the drugs and the sleaze. For years, seemingly kind and wealthy men had given her a taste of the good life, promising the world to her. And each time, one after the other, they'd thrown her back again.

'To be a saviour is a man's fantasy, right? But men can't follow through. They're all talk.'

Belinda sealed her envelope. Tears quivered on her lashes. She put on her sunglasses.

'Nowadays I play on their fantasies for money. It's all just an act. I play the victim, they play the saviour. That's how it is.'

For a moment I wondered if she played the victim with paramedics too, or if her victimhood was less of an act with us. Her tears looked pretty real to me.

Belinda couldn't even scrape together fifty cents for a postage stamp from her purse, so I gave her the money. Before I could turn away she kissed me goodbye on the cheek.

'Thanks so much, I owe you one,' she said. 'Tell Jerry to have a happy Christmas, won't you? He knows where I'll be.'

When I recount the story to Jerry he gets a pang of pity and wants to go back and give her a hug. But I tell him to let her be, let her do what she has to, let her save her own life.

'You're married with kids,' I remind him. 'Don't get her hopes up.'

Jerry's not the first paramedic I've worked with who has a rescue fantasy. We all probably have one, to some extent. But Belinda doesn't need another knight in shining armour.

As we leave Kings Cross on our way back to Bondi, Jerry points out a building next to a 7-Eleven.

'See that joint?'

I nod.

'Swingers club,' he says.

'How d'you know?'

'Went in there on a job once. Guy passed out. There were people humping all over the place.'

I tell Jerry that a few years back, before I met Kaspia, I worked with a swinger. A paramedic swinger in Newcastle. One afternoon the swinger's wife called the ambulance station and asked to speak to me. She said she'd seen me in uniform up the road at Bakers Delight and thought I looked sexy and wanted to invite me to a daytime party with seven of her middle-aged girlfriends. I'd have to knock on the door wearing nothing but a giant red ribbon. She told me I could do whatever I wanted, with any of them, or all at once.

'Please, please, *please* tell me you went along!' cries Jerry, as if in agony.

I shake my head. 'Couldn't do it. I've got principles, see. There's no way in this world I'll wear a red ribbon.'

Jerry doesn't laugh. He's genuinely incredulous, furious. 'Unbelievable! Wait till I tell John about this,' he says. 'That'll get him talking again. He'll give you a bloody hiding for missing out on a good old-fashioned orgy. For crying out loud, what were you thinking?'

★

We reach the Junction and Jerry suggests we go by John's place on our way back to the station. We'd planned to do this anyway, but now Jerry has some gossip to make John laugh there's all the more reason.

I've hesitated dropping in on John till now. Perhaps I should have visited on Christmas Day, and I almost did last week. But what if *he* didn't want to see *me*? I respect people's privacy. Lately, John hasn't been welcoming to social offers from even his closest of friends, and I don't force myself on anyone. Since splitting with Kaspia I've taken up the hermit life myself; I know how it is. Turning up with Jerry doesn't feel as weird or intrusive.

The apartment's on the ground floor of a nondescript unit block. In the stairwell there's a low shelf, a communal library stocked with large-print books; a clue to the age demographic of the other tenants.

'A foyer library should be warning enough to anyone without a walking stick thinking of moving in,' jokes Jerry.

I'm about to knock on the door but Jerry stops me.

'Wait. Let's creep to the front window, see if we can startle John naked or doing something embarrassing, okay?'

That scenario is precisely why I didn't want to come uninvited. I doubt John will be up for Jerry's schoolboy shenanigans. But I reluctantly follow my partner outside and into a garden of thick hydrangeas.

Against the window we cup our hands over our eyes and peer through the glass. Between venetian slats we can see John sunk into a lounge, watching TV. It looks like another repeat of *Dancing with the Stars*. He must have heard us, because without turning his head he calls out, 'Stop fucking around, will you? Front door's open.'

We let ourselves in and John greets us from where he lies. He doesn't get up. The place is a mess. The odour of stale beer and cheap wine lingers under the sickly sweet scented candles burning on the mantelpiece.

'Nice,' I say, nodding to the candles.

'Love Candles,' says John. 'That's what's written on the packet. Good for nothing.'

'Come on, John,' says Jerry with a chuckle. 'You've never had a problem in the love department. Who're you kidding?'

John sighs. 'Yeah, well, there's only one lover I'm interested in and he's fucked off, hasn't he.'

'Guess there's no point telling you that Ben here denied himself an orgy in Newcastle once.'

'You did?' John asks.

I nod. 'They wanted to put a ribbon on me.'

'Like a pageant queen.'

'Exactly. So I objected.'

'Fair enough,' says John, much to Jerry's disappointment. Then he asks if we want some beers.

Jerry points to the crates of empty bottles in a corner by the kitchen. 'Looks like you've drunk them all already,' he says. 'That's gotta be, like, fifty empties right there.'

'Want to bring me another case? Just pile it up on the stretcher like Ben and I did.'

'I don't remember that I did that.'

'You watched me, that's guilty enough.'

He's pleased to see us, but he doesn't look well. He seems lethargic and his face is drawn. I wonder how many visitors he's had since his breakup with Antonio. Jerry reckons not many. People think flamboyant men like John are never short of friends. They always have a party to be at. It's easy to underestimate his loneliness, and it looks to me like he's been on the lounge for days. John has skipped his gym sessions for a fortnight, he says. It's the height of summer and he loves swimming too, but hasn't been in the water since he did laps at Clovelly a few weeks back with Jerry.

'We'll come round after work on Tuesday, if you like,' Jerry says to John. 'I'll bring those beers.' Beer might not be the ideal drink for depressed men to bond over. But if having beers allows John some company, so be it.

'Sure,' says John, 'whatever. Just call me.'

He sounds noncommittal. And calling him hasn't proven very successful to date.

I hear our control on the radio giving us an urgent call in Waterloo, an overdose. John hears it too. He shakes his head.

'Fucking Waterloo,' he says, pressing play on the repeat of *Dancing with the Stars*.

'Go easy on those dancing celebrities, will you?' Jerry says as we bid our farewell.

'Dancing celebrities are all I've got,' John replies. 'Pull the door shut behind you.'

In the hallway, a nosy old woman peeking through the crack of her front door sticks her head out and asks if everything's fine. It's gossip-fishing most likely, rather than neighbourly concern.

'Saw the uniforms, hope the guy's all right,' she says.

'All good,' I reply.

But as we walk away, I'm not so sure.

Lisa, an emergency nurse and one of John's closest friends, is doing a rotation on the triage desk at Sydney Hospital. We see her when we drop off a patient and Jerry tells her how we visited John earlier and found him sitting on his own, watching TV on a sunny day.

'He's really out of sorts,' she says. 'He was up at St Vinnies yesterday, you know, getting seen by a psych registrar.'

No, we didn't know that. Why wouldn't he tell us? Did he feel ashamed about wanting help? Was he worried we'd see him as weak or troubled? Lisa says John's sister had called him and insisted he go to hospital, refusing to take no for an answer. Lisa then met him out the back of Emergency and helped him slip through a fire door like a celebrity, like his idol Heath Ledger might've done.

'Did he come in disguise?' Jerry wants to know.

'Sunglasses,' she replies.

It's a shame that seeing a counsellor is still a dirty secret for many of us. Once, when I had a few sessions at a corporate counselling service, I bumped into a high-ranking paramedic manager in the waiting room. It was such an awkward encounter that for several years afterwards neither of us could look the other in the eye. It shouldn't be this way. I know that, and I also know it's shifting, too slowly perhaps, but workplace cultures don't change overnight.

'Did he stay long?' asks Jerry.

'Not long. He got assessed and went home.'

Lisa went on to say that John seemed pretty wrecked, but he didn't want to stay. The psych registrar wouldn't keep him, anyway. While John was clearly depressed, the doctor felt he wasn't an 'acute risk' to himself.

'Getting pissed in the middle of the day and watching *Dancing with the Stars* on repeat sounds pretty acute to me,' says Jerry.

Lisa shrugs. 'Plenty of blokes do that, you'd be surprised. Besides, I'm not the doctor. What do I know.' She got John to the hospital, and that's an achievement.

A man raps on Lisa's triage window and barks, 'Hey, you! Nurse! I need some fucking help here. My tooth's killing me!'

We leave her with the toothache and go out to the ambulance. It's knock-off time, but the ten-minute drive to Bondi station is always a gamble. Even on overtime, if someone collapses and we're the nearest resource, we'll get the job. Heading back at the end of the day is just about the fastest we ever drive when we're not on a mercy dash.

CHAPTER 14

Jerry and I take our coffees to the beach and chat to the lifeguards starting their shift. The swell is up at the southern end and dozens of surfers are competing for waves. Soft-sand runners ply their route by the sea wall where a couple of artists, up early, are working on a mural. A yoga session is taking place by the shoreline, near a man who's fishing off the beach. On the boulevard in front of us a family of Sikhs walks past, followed by a model who one of the lifeguards thinks is famous, then a couple of Hasidic Jews and an old man with a parrot on his shoulder. This diverse beauty of Bondi is why I love the place, why it's hard for me to leave.

At 8.30 am we get called to an intoxicated male, an Irishman in a backstreet. Nine out of ten times that we're called to a drunk in daylight hours down here it'll be for an Irishman.

Most citizens of Bondi are unaware there are Irish ghettoes in their suburb. A unit block on Simpson Street is one such place. There's a flat there with a missing front door, the rooms inside lined with mattresses on which dozens of backpackers sleep packed together for a fiver a night.

'Where am I?' the Irishman asks, rolling over on the footpath.

'Dublin,' says Jerry in an Irish accent.

The guy looks around, confused. 'Ye shoor aboot dat? What pert a Dublin?'

We give him a lift to his hostel and put him to bed.

Later in the morning we're driving through Vaucluse on the way back from a case when Jerry shouts, 'Stop the ambulance! Quick!'

I brake and pull over. 'What is it?'

Jerry opens his passenger door and gets out. In my mirror I see him walk ten metres back to some junk on the side of the road that looks like it's there for the next council clean-up. Vaucluse is one of the richest suburbs in the country and there are people in vans who make a living by just picking up stuff here that people throw out.

When my partner comes back he is carrying a canvas, at least one by two metres, a painting I can't see until he turns it around and holds it up to show me.

It's a nude. A slightly bored-looking woman with a narrow waist and broad hips.

He lowers the painting and beams. Once Jerry saw the sketch of a nude on an old lady's wall and studied it for ages, until she told him to take it as a gift. But this one, he reckons, is bound for the station.

Jerry puts the nude in the back of the ambulance and we go down New South Head Road. We're halfway to the station when a call comes in for an old man fallen in Point Piper.

'Damn it!' says Jerry.

'Let's turf the nude,' I say.

Jerry looks at me, incredulous. 'Turf the nude? You crazy? We can't do that! She's a beauty, and worth a bit too.'

'Worth a bit too? How do you know?'

'Price tag on the back says $800.'

'That's not much.'

'What do you mean? We just got an $800 painting for nothing! It's going in the gallery.'

'Gallery?'

'Gallery! Ambulance station gallery, right beside *The Gilmour* and that one of Don Quixote. Now drive the bloody ambulance!'

I pick up speed along the bay, where million-dollar yachts are moored, and turn right past the police station. We arrive at the address a short time later.

Jerry and I are hoping the man will just need to be lifted off the ground, but he ends up needing more than that. His name is Harold and he may have been unconscious. He doesn't know what day it is, so he needs a full assessment at the hospital. Luckily, Harold's confused enough to think nothing of it when Jerry puts him into the ambulance beside our nude, her bosom inches from his face.

'Oh, my! How lovely!' the old man remarks with a smile, and he perks right up.

When we finally get the painting to Bondi, Jerry hangs it on the wall of the station and stands back, looking at it as proudly as if he'd painted it himself.

'Mighty fine work,' he says, nodding.

On closer inspection it isn't too bad. Better than the rest of the art on the walls, that's for sure.

The station phone rings and I expect it to be a manager alerting us to a complaint received from the public about a pair of paramedics seen loading up a nude from a Vaucluse council clean-up. But it's only our controller with a job for us in Dover Heights. I breathe a sigh of relief.

It's a mystery call, another 'concern for welfare' case. An elderly woman, Gladys, was meant to be meeting her friends for lunch but didn't show up. They're worried because her husband of fifty years died last week and the funeral was yesterday. We suspect our patient has simply double-booked or forgotten her appointment. But the man who was hanging behind his door is too fresh in our minds for us to be complacent.

There's no answer when Jerry rings the bell of the brick veneer home, which is dwarfed on either side by box-like mansions. Jerry is about to return to the ambulance when I try the doorhandle and find it unlocked.

'Let's check inside,' I say.

Jerry follows me in. I shout, 'Hello? Ambulance here!'

'You're not an ambulance,' Jerry says.

'Very observant,' I reply. 'You check the back room, I'll check the front.'

I don't expect to find anything, so I'm caught off guard when I do. The bedroom is a bloodbath. The woman we're looking for is on the floor, slumped against her dressing table, and she looks deceased.

'Jerry!' I call out. Then, 'Gladys? Gladys, can you hear me?'

Crouching down, I feel for a pulse in her neck. I'm surprised to find she has one. It's weak, and fast. Her chest suddenly heaves with a breath, then she opens her eyes, slowly, like her eyelids are heavy.

Behind me Jerry says, 'Bloody hell,' and goes to get some gear. He calls for backup on his way out the door.

The patient is pale as talcum, and isn't speaking. She smells of alcohol; an empty bottle of sherry lies beside her. She has a large gash on her head from falling against the dresser. It's where she's lost all the blood from. I'm glad I'm wearing gloves.

I lay Gladys flat and raise her legs. Jerry's at my side now, unzipping the red kit of dressings. He holds a trauma pad firmly on Gladys's head, then wraps a roller bandage round it. I can't palpate a blood pressure, meaning she's almost bled out and is hypovolaemic.

Jerry gives Gladys oxygen while I start an IV and an infusion of Hartmann's solution to make up for the blood loss. We need to raise her pressure. Once the line's connected I pump the fluid through, then hang the bag on the handle of a drawer so I can go for a second IV. Jerry leaves to set up the stretcher. By the time he comes back, our patient's more alert. Gladys stares at us and in a feeble voice she asks, 'Are you angels?'

'Hardly,' Jerry snorts.

'Am I still alive?'

'Yes, you are,' I say.

Gladys looks downcast.

'But I wanted to be with my husband,' she says.

I stop pushing the infusion and glance over at Jerry. His face is as solemn as mine.

'I'm sorry,' I say.

*

The sadness we feel about Gladys slows us down for the rest of the day. But we have to leave work on a high, and Jerry does his best to lighten things up. Our final patient is a woman with emphysema who needs some oxygen. When I open our oxygen kit I'm horrified to see a banana skin lying there among the masks and tubes.

I mouth a swearword to Jerry and he gives a cheeky smile. He knows how much I hate the smell of bananas, how I can't be in the ambulance when he's eating one, how banana skins make me nauseous. A banana skin in the oxygen kit is a deliberate act of sabotage and it's not the first time he's done it. Last year, Jerry secretly put a banana skin under the driver's seat of the ambulance in the height of summer without telling me. The smell drove me crazy until I searched high and low and discovered it there. Everyone at the station thought it was hilarious.

As we sign in to the ambulance's data terminal the following night I remember it's the date of Kaspia's show. It would be easy for me to drop by in the ambulance on the pretext of a call. Jerry, with his appreciation of nudes, would love the burlesque too; he's been to several shows already and delights in the nipple-tassel-twirling. But there's a good chance Kaspia might see us in the shadows. And if she didn't then our friend Russall, the director, would. A casual visit could backfire and mess up any chance I have of getting back together with her.

If I'm honest with myself, visiting the club wouldn't really be about catching a glimpse of Kaspia again. It would be to see if any handsome men in the audience, impressed with her performance, were buying her drinks and trying to seduce her. I would be there for no good reason. Kaspia and I had never made an explicit vow of celibacy for our time of separation; it was just implied that we wouldn't sleep with others. I guess we should have discussed the parameters of our breakup, the finer details. We should have been clear, to prevent these distrustful, shameful thoughts arising.

By 10 pm the city has half a dozen emergencies waiting for an ambulance. We're sent into town and get one right away, a stabbing near Kings Cross Station. On the way I tell Jerry about a stabbing I went to earlier in the year outside a night-club in the city. A man was standing on the street, looking at us expectantly when we pulled up, so I asked him if he knew where the patient was. He replied, 'Right here.' Then he turned around to show us the handle of a kitchen knife sticking out of his back.

On Victoria Street, a flock of women dressed as nurses are heading to a costume party. As Jerry and I fly past they kick up their Barbie-doll legs in our headlights and swing toy stethoscopes in the air.

'Check my heart!' Jerry shouts from his open window, but he's barely audible over the siren. His bravado tonight is extreme and I'm pretty sure I know the reason. Earlier on, when we stopped to refuel at a Caltex, he visited the toilet and returned with a mischievous grin.

'Smell anything?' he asked me.

'No. What?'

He leaned across and pulled his collar down, exposing his neck. 'Go on, take a sniff.'

I did, but still couldn't smell anything.

'What is it?' I asked him.

'There was a vending machine in the toilets dispensing pheromone wipes. Passion Wipes, they're called. I've always been curious. So I put a coin in and got one and dabbed it on myself.'

No wonder he's been acting like he's irresistible. I can only see it leading to trouble. He's the friskiest married man I know, even without the aid of Passion Wipes.

When we arrive at the scene, the cops direct us to a man lying on his back with two stab wounds to his abdomen. The footpath is crammed with people, but no one saw anything, or so they say. It's crowded, and a passing drunk trips over our stab victim and lands on his face. Others stand about, filming the victim with their mobile phones, laughing at the spectacle like it somehow isn't real for them.

Jerry pulls the stretcher out of the ambulance straightaway, setting up for a 'load and go'. It's the best approach in a major trauma. I remember Jerry's story about sticking his finger in a guy's heart and whisking the patient off, saving his life. Now I'll have just *one* minute, in the back of the ambulance between Kings Cross and St Vincent's, to examine the patient for other stab wounds, to connect the oxygen, to auscultate lungs, to do a blood pressure, to attach the monitor, to get an IV and to set up fluids. All this can be achieved, of course, but it's a juggle. More difficult to manage are the other intoxicated punters who get in our way and slap me on the shoulder and ask, 'Oi, ambo, what the fuck happened?' as if we have the time to stop and satisfy their morbid curiosity while trying to save a man bleeding to death.

Friday and Saturday nights can be enjoyable for a short while around midnight, about halfway through the shift. That's the time we'll find ourselves pushing through dense and pumping dance floors to reach our patients, with revellers grinding up against us in the hope we'll drop our gear and join the fun. But that peak is quickly over. By 3 am the streets are ugly. Drunk men kick over bins for no good reason and stumble onto the road, oblivious to traffic. Women carry their high heels and walk barefoot in crooked lines down filthy pavements or sit in the gutter, crying about bad boyfriends while waiting for taxis that never show up. Fights, sometimes brawls, break out at regular intervals. And that's what we're called to next, a brawl on Darlinghurst Road.

We arrive in the middle of it: men grappling and punching each other while girlfriends do their best to drag them off. Jerry flicks on the siren to try to disperse them, but none of them cares. We can tell by their haircuts they're not from the city or the eastern suburbs. Like many of our customers on Friday and Saturday nights, they've come into town from the suburbs out west.

A man dumps his semiconscious friend at the front of the ambulance. He bangs his fist on the bonnet and yells, 'Don't just sit there, dickheads! Look at this guy!'

Where are the police? Tied up at another assault, no doubt.

We open our doors and get out to treat the patient. But our ambulance is quickly overrun by souped-up brawlers. They climb into the back, their faces sprayed with blood, demanding to be treated. Five patients are on the stretcher, spitting teeth onto the floor. I lock the doors to stop any more from getting in and call for a second ambulance.

There are few older paramedics left in the inner city. Some shifts now, I look around and realise I'm the longest-serving officer on duty. Most of the others have wisely escaped long ago to the suburbs or up the coast to country towns. Ask them why and most will mention they got fed up with the never-ending barrage of abusive, alcohol-affected patients. I often wonder why I'm still here when I know how unhealthy it is in the long term. It's not that I'm addicted to the danger and adrenalin, more that I'm drawn to the craziness of humanity pressed together in the city, the horror and the beauty of it. I'm drawn to people, to observing the wonders of our species in a concentrated setting.

Until I'm caught up in a brawl, that is.

Jerry's pheromone scent has not been working well for him. Nurses at the hospital seem to pay him less attention than usual, and he's not happy about it.

'Cost me two dollars,' he complains, shaking his head.

Then, at 4 am, it finally takes effect. Our patient, Ethel, is an eighty-year-old woman who can't control her bowels. This, it turns out, is not the only thing the old duck can't control. Poor Jerry. She can't keep her hands off him. Ethel tells us she used to be an accordionist who travelled the countryside playing in roadside pubs. But tonight her hands are playing Jerry's leg as he tries to do his paperwork beside her in the ambulance.

'Now, now, dear,' says Jerry, trying to calm her down.

'Oh, Jerry!' Ethel coos. 'How about I take you home and we make love all night? What do you say? Forget about the hospital. Turn this ambulance round and take me home again, will you? Or we could get a room. Yes, what a fabulous idea. Shall we get a room? Let's get a room!'

I angle the rear-vision mirror down a little and see my partner squirming around, trying his best to politely fend off her prying fingers. Ethel's got him backed right up in the corner of his seat and is reaching for his crotch.

'Madam, we're not permitted to make love with our patients,' he tells her.

Jerry climbs awkwardly over the treatment console and into the front cabin to escape her. Then he reaches for a box of tissues, pulls a few out and starts feverishly rubbing his neck and wrists, trying to remove the remnants of his service-station Passion Wipes.

We've been up all night without a break, and if not for the heat and Jerry's hilarious antics I wouldn't be so alert. But as we head to Maroubra to treat an unconscious man, the creeping weight of fatigue descends on me. Before we're out of Kensington, Jerry's fast asleep against his window and I'm drawing on every bit of willpower to stay awake. A giant copper-coloured moon hangs above the suburbs and gives me strength.

Pulling into the street, I catch sight of police red-and-blues and I nudge Jerry. He opens his eyes and yawns.

Our patient is lying on someone's front lawn. He's built like a rugby player. It seems to us a simple case of intoxication. But the man doesn't budge when we shake him. None of our painful stimuli work, and I'm reluctant to try too many arm pinches on account of the last experience.

Jerry and I decide to load the guy up with the help of two cops and let him keep snoring. The police drive behind us to hospital as they have some other business there, and we're grateful they do. At a set of lights, without the slightest warning, our patient awakes with a jolt. Unlike the usual slow and bewildered regaining of consciousness we usually see, the man switches on like a floodlight, and he's angry.

In the rear-vision mirror I see his fist lash out and strike Jerry in the face. Jerry tries defending himself but the guy is too big. He swings again and Jerry ducks. I slam my foot on the brake and halt in the middle of the road, then press the duress button on our dash. I switch on the flashing lights and jump out. At the rear of the ambulance I wave to the cops, but they've already seen the ambulance rocking and are running over. I fling the back doors open and see our patient pinning Jerry to the treatment seat with one leg, and kicking him with the other.

The two policemen dive into the ambulance and pounce on the man, but he throws them off with a beast-like strength. His feet and fists pummel the air, striking out at anything. The cops try again, just as police reinforcements screech round the corner and another three cops bundle in. A minute later five police have the man restrained.

I find Jerry ambling in a stupor down the middle of Anzac Parade. His uniform is torn and bloodied, his hair all over the place, his shirt hanging out of his trousers. While the police handcuff our patient and put him in a cage truck I guide Jerry to the passenger seat of the ambulance. I check his wounds then drive him to hospital.

Jerry stares blankly ahead. 'I was just sitting there,' he murmurs. 'I didn't do a thing.'

But aggression isn't always provoked. Patients can wake up like this: confused, disorientated, violent. Waking the unresponsive is a roll of the dice. Who knows what nightmare we're dragging them out of. And if they wake in our ambulance we've got nowhere to run. We're trapped in a cage with a tiger. A friendly face and a soothing voice work wonders, but there's no guarantee. If a paramedic as jovial and charming as Jerry gets flogged, none of us is safe.

Once Jerry's been checked by a doctor he takes the rest of the shift off. There's only a few hours left of it, anyway. 'I've had enough of this bullshit,' he says. I can tell that he means it. An hour earlier we were laughing hysterically about Ethel's advances – now this. Sometimes even our comedy won't shield us from the onslaught of violence.

I drive Jerry back to the ambulance station and help him get his stuff together. Then I give him a handshake and tell him I'll call him tomorrow.

After leaving work I do something terribly stupid. I'm exhausted, delirious, not thinking straight. And even though I curse myself, I can't stop.

I drive to Kaspia's place in Balmain.

Before I know it I'm in the Cross City Tunnel then over the Anzac Bridge and taking the turn-off to Mullens Street. The suburb is quiet; it's 7 am after a Friday night and people are sleeping in. I park just down from Balmain Town Hall and walk the rest of the way. I go up the stone steps to her terrace on the ridge. I'm not sure why I'm here or what I plan to do.

The front door is closed, and I can't hear anything when I put my ear against it. Then I go to the window next to the door. The bamboo blind is up, and I peer into the room. When I'm sure that Kaspia isn't in there I put my face to the glass and have a better look. The room is nicely decorated; she's very good at that. Then I see something on the floor near the hatstand that makes me sick. It punches me in the guts as hard as I've ever been hit.

Lying there, as if thrown off hastily in passion, is a pair of male boots.

CHAPTER 15

I'm stunned. My heart pounds in anguish and anger, my head races with thoughts: how could I have been so mistaken? How quickly I dismissed John's pessimism, the reality checks he always tried to give me. Suddenly, with a pair of male boots, my assumptions have collapsed. This isn't how things were meant to pan out. Our separation wasn't intended as an opportunity for us to sleep with other people. We separated to experience life apart, to give us space to ponder, to reflect on the relationship from the outside in. But what if I'd misunderstood all along?

I drive away with tears on my face, barely able to keep my car on the road. I've been awake for twenty-six hours. It feels like I've endured a lifetime of drama in the space of a day and a night.

★

Back in my apartment I pour a bowl of cereal but decide I don't feel hungry. I leave it in the sink and take a shower. Then I fall on the bed like a tree cut down. My breathing is shallow and it feels like I haven't exhaled the breath that I took back at Kaspia's window.

The truth is, I've blown it. I was doubtful, indecisive, neglectful in our relationship. Kaspia suggested the split, but I'd driven her to it. In the months before we separated, Kaspia and I were talking about marriage and kids. I told her I wasn't ready for either, but realise now that's not what a partner wants to hear after a decade together. While Kaspia never said it, I know my lack of commitment was part of why she wanted to separate. At the very least, I suppose, to see if I could hack a life without her.

Even as we packed our stuff into separate boxes, I didn't protest. The break never felt permanent because I told myself it wasn't, but maybe in her mind it was.

I roll out of bed and go to my cupboard. I find a scarf: silk, paisley print. It's one of Kaspia's that I packed by mistake. I go down the stairs and loop it round the banister. I'm not good with knots, but I know what'll work.

Then I hear my own voice talking me down.

Stop! Look what you're doing. This is forever! Think about that. Think about your mother . . .

I think about my mother getting the news from the cops who come to her door. The tears come again and I reach for my phone to call my folks. My mother answers and I try to sound normal, like there's nothing wrong, but she knows, she can tell, that there's something not right. She says, 'Hold on, we're coming over. Don't do anything till we get there, okay?' She knows, as my father does, what I'm capable of.

I take down the scarf and fold it away. I could never let Mum see it there.

My parents arrive. They want to know what's going on, but I refuse to talk specifics. I just tell them I hate the silence, that I miss my life with Kaspia.

They stay all afternoon and beg me not to work. Take the next shift off, they say – the week, the month. But what's my other option? To bum around and wallow in self-pity? To use up all my sick leave till I get an official letter putting me on notice? My parents worry I'll be tired, that I'll make foolish choices. But my love for them is endless and I realised the moment I was hanging up that scarf that I couldn't put them through such grief. I also know there's beauty in this life, even if at times we're blind to it, like the New Year's fireworks behind an overpass. The inner voice that talked me down is using all the classic lines I've used on others. Being on the receiving end, I see how I *do* sound 'a little bit Oprah', as my patient Courtney pointed out. But these talk-down clichés are what I now grasp onto. They're small but solid footholds.

My parents insist I stay at their house for a couple of days. None of us mentions it, but we all know it's suicide watch. I reluctantly agree. I can leave for work from there.

At the home I grew up in there is safety and love, but it also feels like I've come full circle, like I've failed at life. As if my shot at being an adult didn't work out and here I am, a child again. I promise myself I won't stay for long.

When I wake up after two hours to get ready for work I know I've paid only a fraction of my sleep debt. My palms ache and my fingers are stiff. It's a sign I've been clenching my fists in my sleep again. I've been doing it for years now, long before Kaspia and I moved apart. I think it's the job, the shift work, the city. I get palpations too, every now and then.

I shave, take a shower and drive to the station. The world outside seems slightly blurry, like a poorly filmed flashback in a poorly made movie.

Down at the station I team up with another Bondi paramedic just back from annual leave. Her name's Donna and she's filling in for Matt. Donna's been around awhile and has a reputation as a good clinician. She could have studied medicine, become a doctor. But she loves the streets like I do, and in this country doctors don't work on ambulances. She rolls her own cigarettes, smokes as hard as Barry. She likes to be called Sydway, after the street directory, because she reckons she never has to look up an address. And she's pretty good, I admit, although I've caught her more than once having a peek at the directory, at which time she'll say she's just 'confirming' that she's right.

Our shift starts slow, and for once I wish it wouldn't. I want to get moving, I want the distraction. I want to announce to the suburb that I'm ready for action.

We're sent to a girl at a barbecue who's throwing up cheap wine. She's been drinking since 10 am and now she's on her hands and knees, spitting and drooling.

'Oh my God, I'm so sick! I don't know what's wrong with me . . . I just don't understand.'

When I politely suggest she's vomiting because she might've had too much booze she loses her temper.

'I'm not fucking drunk, you fucking arsehole! Are you calling me drunk? I only had some champagne, three rums, and two shots, for fuck's sake!' Then she clutches her friend's leg and cries, 'Get him away from me. Get him away!'

Donna watches from a distance, letting me solve my own problems.

It hurts to grovel, but the patient's always right. So I ask her to forgive me for suggesting she might be intoxicated and she softens enough to accept a lift home. There are plenty of temptations for an argument in this job. And even though I've learnt the hard way not to bite, I still get myself in trouble for it now and then.

★

We take a patient from one hospital to another, then we treat a man with cellulitis and one with trouble urinating. The cases are banal, but as soon as I'm chatting to my patients I'm in their lives and not in mine, and that is what I'm here for.

Sometime after midnight we're sent to a Vietnam War veteran, Richard. He phoned one of his friends and hinted at suicide, so his friend called an ambulance.

Richard's front door is already open, and we go in to find him penning the lines of a suicide note. He stops and looks up.

'Bloody hell! Karl called you, didn't he? Bastard! The deed would be done by now if I had a gun.'

He puts down his pen and begins reading aloud his unfinished suicide note. Donna and I pull up chairs and sit at the table and listen. It's often like this, our patients presenting their innermost feelings without hesitation, as if they've known us a lifetime. The least we can do is spare them our ears.

'I did things in the war, things I can't live with anymore. There are things I can't talk about, things I'm not allowed to. But now that I'm dead it's time you all knew. It was a covert operation on a Saturday morning in Saigon. I was in a café and I shot a woman dead, single shot to the head. She was going to blow the place up; least, that's what I thought when she came through the doors. Turned out I was wrong. She never had a bomb, never had one at all.'

He stops for a moment, his faced clenched up. A tear drops on the page, smudges the ink.

'Jan, you're wonderful, you've been great in my life, same with Terry and the kids. You put up with my nightmares and moods, and I'm sorry for that. I understand why you divorced me. And I'm glad we stayed friends. But Norm, you let me down, and you, Tom, you did too.'

Richard looks up, lowers the page.

'That's where I got to when you ambos came in. What d'you think?'

'Why don't you finish it, Richard?' I say. 'Finish and send it. Mail it tomorrow when the post office opens.' Then I think of a line John loves to use. *You don't need to take your life to make people listen.*

Richard nods and agrees to come with us. As we drive him up to the hospital for counselling, I think of John's words about making people listen. I hadn't thought of writing a note when I was standing at the banister earlier in the day. It never occurred to me. Using Kaspia's scarf would've said enough, I'm sure. But why say something in death that can be said in life? What's the point in Kaspia finding out how much I really love her only once I'm dead and gone? She needs to know it *now.* She needs to know that I want to make a life with her, that our separation has beaten me. I want her to forgive me for my carelessness with what we had.

After my night shift I stay in bed and sleep until midday. I wake to the smell of my favourite soup and the sound of my brothers and sister in the kitchen. My parents must have told them I was doing it tough and invited them for lunch. Their concern is appreciated, but all I want to do is eat and go back to bed. I could sleep for a week, the way I feel now. The emotion of yesterday, on top of the shiftwork and sleep deprivation, has left me exhausted.

The person I really want to talk to is Kaspia; I don't care about the agreement. But I have to be rested and clear-minded for that, and I don't feel either of those things right now.

I stay another night at my parents' house, then tell them I'm feeling more positive and drive back to mine. I may be in a better place emotionally, but my energy's sapped. I feel like I've picked up a virus, maybe from one of my patients. So much for the paramedic's super-immunity.

Late on Friday morning on the eleventh of January, I'm woken by a phone call. I see it's Jerry. Damn it! Didn't I promise to call him to see how he was going after our patient beat him up? Consumed by my own emotional crisis, I haven't been looking anywhere but inward. I feel selfish and guilty.

'So sorry, Jerry, I meant to call you. How are you?'

But Jerry ignores me. His tone is flat and serious. Is he still in shock from his assault?

'Did I wake you?' he asks.

'Yeah, but no worries. You okay?'

Jerry clears his throat.

'I'm really sorry to tell you this, but it looks like John went off The Gap late yesterday.'

I'm silent for a moment, not sure if I heard him right.

'What do you mean?'

'They found John's car near the lookout. People saw a man go over. He landed on the rocks and a wave washed him out. There's no body yet, but we're pretty sure it was him.'

I can't talk, can't reply. I hang up the phone and get off the bed. The room is spinning. My breathing quickens and my heart thuds like it wants to escape. I walk in circles, gripped by anger. Then a surge of grief crashes over me. I don't know what to do.

A few minutes later I pick up the phone and call Trevor, the area supervisor, to get more information. Like so many relatives I've broken bad news to, I feel as if I'm inside a dream, a nightmare. I need someone else to confirm it.

But I'm choked up and Trevor has trouble understanding me.

'Okay, buddy, I can hear you're upset, I'm staying on the line until you're ready. Take your time. I've been on the phone all morning with other people crying too. Are you there?'

When I manage to get some words out I ask Trevor what happened. He confirms that witnesses saw John fall from The Gap, after which the police found his car in the no-stopping zone. He'd left it unlocked, his wallet with paramedic ID on the dash. An ambulance crew from Randwick was passing by and the police hailed them down and asked the paramedics if they knew the officer the wallet belonged to. Everyone in the area knows John well, loves and respects him. The two paramedics were understandably distressed by the sudden realisation of what must have happened.

'Listen,' says Trevor, 'I'm sending a peer support officer over. She won't be long. Sit tight.'

I pace around for a while until I calm down enough to phone Jerry back. He tells me police helicopters have been circling Watsons Bay all morning. Unfortunately the winds are high, the ocean churned up, the waves eight foot. The weather is rotten for aerial searches. But the police are carrying on in the riskiest of conditions.

'We openly talked about suicide,' says Jerry. 'He told me he'd never do it.'

Recipients of tragic news are often numb and distant. I feel detached from everything around me now, as I try to grasp this turn of events, how it came to pass, how we all could have missed it.

John was displaying unmistakable signs of depression, but after his nephew took his own life, after seeing how hard the death was for his sister and parents, John swore he'd never put them through his own suicide. I can only imagine that all rational thought must have left him in the hours before his death, that he spiralled out of control on the afternoon he died, an afternoon when I was sleeping.

Barely a fortnight has passed since I last worked with John. Even though I was his paramedic partner at the beginning of his breakup with Antonio, even though I listened to him share his troubles with me before he shut himself away, like Jerry I never thought he would take his life. He went on helping strangers with their burdens at work, despite his own hardships. He could pick others up, but not himself. He'd counsel the depressed and suicidal with compassion, yet tell me in private he wished they'd 'pull themselves together and quit complaining'. Perhaps it's also what he said to himself, what many of us say to ourselves, quietly, on the inside. *Pull yourself together, quit complaining.* Why else are we so bad at seeking help? And what happens when we *can't* pull ourselves together anymore, but won't ask for help? What then?

This?

The peer support officer who knocks at my door is Mandy from the train job. I'm relieved it's her because she's kind, and we've always clicked.

'Did you get the chewy off your pants?' I ask.

'Eventually,' she replies, smiling. She gives me a hug and I make her a cup of tea, and we sit together on my balcony and look at the cloudy skyline over the city.

'How are the others?'

She goes through the names of everyone at the station, one by one, as well as those who've recently left. Mandy tells me Donna's inconsolable and is spending time with Antonio. Tracy collapsed on hearing the news, but she's all right now. Matt couldn't stop swearing. Others cried or hung up after finding out and haven't been reachable since.

'I'll be visiting quite a few people today,' she says.

Mandy was a friend of John's too, and I suddenly feel bad it's me being counselled. But she's here in uniform, professionally, putting her own grief on hold to support the rest of us.

'If only he'd called me,' I tell her. 'He asked *me* to call *him* and every time I did, his phone went to message bank and he'd never ring back.'

A depressed person, let alone a depressed paramedic, is not good at reaching out. They're much better at pushing away.

'He *did* go to St Vincent's a couple of times,' she says, confirming what Lisa, his nurse friend, had told us. 'They knew he was in a dark place, but he never alluded to suicide. He knew the proper things to say, right? He was smart, he could lie. Everyone's shocked.'

John's the seventh paramedic I've worked with whose life has ended this way.

Mandy says the Health Minister is well aware of the concerning rates of suicide in the industry. But what can be done? No one understands how we work, and the impact the work has on us. We're like a counterculture, living on the fringes. Most other city folk go about their days and nights oblivious to the suffering, the psychological and social crises we engage with. From where we stand, our view of the world is pretty bleak. Black comedy and camaraderie sustain us for a while; so too does the easing of our patients' pain. But the stress accumulates. We harden ourselves to the trauma, we harden the fuck up, but in doing so become hardened to ourselves. The high walls we have built for protection can block our emotional expression. They keep our suffering on the inside, and when something goes wrong, some of us implode.

It's time to call Kaspia, to break the agreement. I need to talk. Life's too short, too fragile not to act. I don't care about those boots I saw in her house, a man's boots. Kaspia has the right to do what she pleases, as do I, if I wanted to. But in the wake of John's death, our uncertain relationship status doesn't seem so important. She's the one I can talk to, the one I've always talked to, with a heart the whole world could fit into.

She answers my call immediately.

'Hello?'

'It's me.'

'I know. You okay?'

'Yeah, I'm sorry to call.'

'It's fine.'

I'm relieved she doesn't sound angry that I've broken our pact. I ask her how her show went and she says it was a sellout, a real hit with the crowd.

She asks me how my Christmas and New Year's was.

'No good without you.'

'Of course you'd say that,' she says with a laugh.

'Happy New Year, by the way.'

'Same to you,' she says. 'Is everything okay? Has something come up?'

She's always had good instincts, Kaspia. She can read my voice as well as my face.

'Yeah. It's John. He took his own life.'

'He what?'

'He took his own life, up at The Gap.'

I can hear her voice breaking. 'Oh, darling . . . I'm sorry.'

'I wish he'd just called me.'

'There's no point in wishing, not now.'

I hear her sadness: for John, for us, for me. Her voice is reassuring, warm and comforting. The love I feel for her blocks the grief out, if only for a moment.

When she invites me over to her place in Balmain I want to say yes, that I'll be there in an hour. But instead the fool in me replies, 'You might have company, a date or something . . .'

'A date or something?'

'Yeah, like you did after your show.' I try to explain, but dig myself deeper: 'I was in the area and wanted to drop in, but saw a bloke's boots through your window.'

'You serious?' she asks me, laughing. 'You didn't recognise the boots? They would've been Russall's!'

Of course: no one wears boots like that in summer except our friend Russall the director. I've seen those boots a hundred times. And in my state the other morning, I'd forgotten that he lives up the coast and crashes in Kaspia's spare room after shows.

I feel the tension in my body dissolve.

'You really aren't thinking straight, are you?' Kaspia says.

'I guess not.'

'So, then, are you coming over?'

It's a tempting offer. But I don't want her to think that I'm using John's death to garner sympathy, or try to win her back. And, as she rightly pointed out, I'm not in the best frame of mind, not yet. So I tell her I'll give her a call, maybe in the next few days.

Our managers are arranging time off for everyone at the station, whoever needs it. But odd as it might seem to others, when my next shift comes round I go back to work. Matt's there too, filling in for Donna. Maybe I've returned because I'm still in disbelief. When I go up the station stairs I see John's pigeonhole full of payslips and letters, and when I go into the change room I touch for a second the cold metal door of his locker. In the lounge area, Trevor is waiting for us with coffees. As with the families we counsel after loved ones die, he patiently answers all of our questions.

'How do you know it was John? How are you sure?'

Trevor says that the witnesses who saw John leave his car described him with precision. After John went over, a tourist on the clifftop somewhat morbidly took a photo of his body on the rocks below, before the waves washed him off. The police were able to examine the picture and show it to Antonio and a couple of John's best friends for identification. When they fully zoomed in, it was unmistakably John, says Trevor. He was lying on his side, in shallow water, a unique tattoo visible on his leg.

'It's only a ten-minute drive to there from his place,' says Matt. 'You're dead in twelve minutes.'

He's right. When caught in the vortex of self-annihilation, it's almost impossible to get out in twelve minutes. Research shows that when people decide to suicide, nearly half of them make an attempt straightaway. We all suspect John was intoxicated too, perhaps making it harder for him to resist the current he was in. His death sounded impulsive rather than planned, but it's hard to be sure.

Suicide deaths nearly always leave behind loved ones wracked with guilt who wonder if they could've done more. The dreaded if-onlys are inevitable. We've heard them a thousand times. *If only I'd come home earlier. If only I'd listened to her. If only I'd answered my phone.* It's a normal reaction, but one usually based on false assumptions, and our appropriate response as paramedics is to tell them they did all they could, that it was out of their control, that it would've happened anyway. We say these things lest their guilt become a crippling affliction. But even if guilt is overcome, the sadness never goes away.

Now it's me who wonders if I did enough for John. At work he was distant, dishevelled, disinterested, as I'd never seem him before. The changes were dramatic, the signs of a man whose strength was fading. I should have known where those signs were headed. I'm trained to know, and I failed to act. Depression is treatable and I didn't do the best I could to connect with him in his final weeks, especially in his final days. I was so caught up in my own world I didn't recognise how much lower he had got. I never considered his depression could be fatal. But heartbreak is a psychological injury, and John was bleeding out.

There's a bunch of flowers on the table in the station courtesy of Rose Bay Police. Matt tells me he accepted the flowers earlier from a junior constable who dropped them over. According to Matt, the constable said, 'Here are the flowers for the guy who topped himself.'

Matt gives a short laugh. 'Can you believe the cop said that? Crazy shit.'

Clearly the officer has more to learn about how to describe suicide and deliver condolences. But we're grateful for the police response, the flowers, and especially the search. The Rose Bay Police have always been our partners at The Gap. It's our tragic meeting place.

'How long was John in the job for?' asks Matt.

I think for a moment. 'Twenty years or so.'

'He would've talked down a heck of a lot of people in that time, wouldn't he?'

'Yeah,' I say. 'Who knows. Eighty? A hundred?'

'Geez,' he says, shaking his head.

For every person who dies at The Gap, many more are persuaded not to. Some by the police or police negotiators, some by paramedics, some by locals like the elderly Don Ritchie, who lives in a house opposite Jacobs Ladder on the southern side, a man known to talk people down then invite them home for tea. I'm confident, in the end, that many of the people John rescued from the edge found hope and love, meaning or redemption, God or enlightenment, happiness or peace, in the land of the living. Some might even remember John, that gentle man who helped them see some reason as they stood at the brink, the point of no return.

But where were we when John was standing there? Our friend, our brother?

Before we pull out for our first job of the night, I can't help thinking about John as another of the many lives I've had a chance to save, but failed to.

*

It doesn't take Matt and me very long to figure out we're not in a state to be working. We're here, but our minds are not. Even my own sadness about Kaspia has been overshadowed by my intensifying grief. I can only imagine what John's family, his parents, brother and sisters are going through right now, and what Antonio must be feeling.

It's raining steadily and we drive staring quietly at the swishing windscreen wipers, lost in thought.

After a while Matt says, 'Donna and some others went up to The Gap earlier today and put flowers on the fence. Tied ribbons to the wire at the place he went over.'

Given John's affection for us, his was perhaps the most considerate method of suicide. Even so, while John might have spared us the trauma of discovering his body, he overlooked the fact that every call to The Gap henceforth will make us think of him.

The controllers go easy on us today, and for that we're grateful. A thirty-six-year-old woman with numb hands; a man with mild back pain; another with an earache. Could a roach have crawled inside? He needs to know. The other night I welcomed non-emergencies as useful distractions, but now the patients grate on me. I'm tempted to share our loss with them, bring perspective to their ingrown toenails.

Then at 3 pm, much to our dismay, we're off to The Gap.

I've never heard a controller so apologetic. 'I can get the Paddington crew to go up there instead,' she offers.

'It's okay, we're closer,' I say.

Matt shakes his head. 'That's fucked,' he says.

But he knows as well as I do that we had the choice of a day off work and we chose to come in. The Gap was always a risk – more than a risk, if the past couple of months was anything to go by.

I drive up there with lights, no siren. I go much faster than I have before. Suddenly this woman threatening to take her life matters ten times more to me than she might have done a week ago, when she would have been another 'Gap job'.

Three police cars are parked in a line, but there's not a cop in sight. We ascend the path to Gap Bluff, which runs between bushes along the top. After a few rocky bends we see a huddle of police around a girl sitting on the safe side of the fence. She has red hair and facial piercings, and the cops have their handcuffs on her, not because she's arrested, but to make it harder for her to get up and run to the cliff. A constable tells me they dragged her away from the edge. She struggles to shake them off, but they grip her arms firmly with black leather gloves.

She yells, 'Why are you doing this? Leave me alone! I was talking to my boyfriend, I was talking on the phone. Can't I sit on the edge and talk to my boyfriend? It's a free world, isn't it. Let go of me – I haven't done anything wrong!'

I ask the cops to un-cuff her. I tell her my name and ask for hers.

'Veronica,' she spits.

'You're not in trouble,' I say. 'We're worried about you, that's all. Are you aware how many people die up here? We're concerned for your safety.'

'Bullshit you're fucking concerned!' she barks.

Just as I'm about to say more I catch sight of a bunch of flowers tied with ribbon to the fence. The flowers are fresh and I realise they're the ones that Donna and the others put there today. When I turn back I lock eyes with the Rose Bay Police inspector, who has come up the path. He has seen me notice the flowers and he quickly averts his gaze.

I ask him, 'This is the spot, isn't it?'

Without lifting his head he answers, 'Yeah, it's the spot. I'm sorry, mate.'

Everyone goes quiet. Matt gets up and walks to the fence and looks out to sea. Perhaps he's thinking he'll catch sight of John, I don't know. Veronica can tell something's up. She frowns and looks around, confused.

'What the hell's going on?' she asks.

The cops don't say anything; they just look at me standing in front of Veronica and then over at Matt. A young police-woman wipes her eye with her sleeve.

'Some people we don't reach in time, Veronica,' I say. 'Some people who we care about, we lose them. But with you we have a chance, understand?'

Veronica doesn't quite know what to make of her highly strung rescuers, of the emotion going round. It's all too weird and she sighs and gives in. We help her to her feet and start down the track to the ambulance.

After work I go to Bondi Beach for a swim. It's dusk, shark feeding time I know, but I don't give a damn. The clouds have disappeared and the waves are merely two foot. The winds that plagued the helicopter's efforts to retrieve John's body have long disappeared. But there's no point searching for our friend anymore. It's a waiting game now, to see if and when his body turns up.

Diving into the ocean at the end of a shift is more than physical purification from the gore and bacteria. It's the purging of sadness, a cleansing of the mind. It's a ritual I rely on to help preserve my sanity. But as I plunge beneath the waves and come up on the other side I find myself gasping in panic, struggling to breathe. What if John were here now, close by? What if his sea-swollen body was tumbling along in one of these waves? What if I came face to face with him under water, his eyes wide open, looking right at me? He could be anywhere around. It wouldn't be the first time a body from The Gap has drifted this far south. The thought is so terrible that my stomach churns and I begin to retch. Then the horror turns to anguish and I shed some tears, until I can't distinguish between the taste of my tears and the taste of the sea.

CHAPTER 16

Two nights in a row I wake in a sweat from fitful sleep, once from a dream in which I was reading John's suicide note. But John never left one of those. The police, along with Antonio and Mick, the paramedic whose house John was staying in, looked high and low, to no avail. I wasn't surprised. John was cynical about suicide notes. He described them once as 'terribly passé', each essentially the same. I always disagreed with him on that point; I've read many, and there's variety enough. There are heartfelt goodbyes, but also notes designed to punish, to heap guilt on those the person feels neglected or wronged them. John might not have left a note, but he left behind plenty of guilt, even for those who loved and supported him. And guilt is the cruellest of punishments. It lingers in unexpected ways, sometimes for years.

As powerful a message as suicide may seem to the deeply despondent, it is tragically flawed if the intention is to punish others. Even if the targets *do* suffer because of it or, less likely, change for the better, how would the departed ever know, or benefit from it? *You don't need to take your life to make people listen*, I wish I'd said to John. The line I'd learnt from him.

Now he's gone, I too feel guilt, but I don't resist it. I sit with it. I reflect on my failings and where I could improve. But I will not punish myself. There's nothing constructive in that.

I share my feelings with Jerry when he arrives back at work. He nods in agreement. We can learn from this sadness, to be vigilant for the signs of depression in friends, to take these signs more seriously and reach out more assertively to those we know will not, or cannot, do it themselves.

'He was pissed off with the world,' says Jerry. 'He shouldn't have allowed one person to bring down his empire, his whole self. A single fucking breakup! He owed it to himself to get past those points, we all do. Get past them and you'll be okay. He should've come for a swim with me, or at least stayed on the fucking lounge. Even time can heal.'

Jerry signs out his restricted medications, then heats up his dinner in the microwave. Any scars from his assault seem well and truly healed, at least the physical ones.

Thousands of city dwellers are still away on vacation and the streets are near deserted. Or so it seems. The poor, the lonely, the homeless and schizophrenic: few of them have holiday houses up the coast or luxury campers for touring in.

'Can't believe they sent you and Matt to The Gap,' Jerry says, shaking his head. 'You should take time off, mate, a week of sick leave. You know what John would say? *Milk it, baby!* If it was one of us who died, you or me for instance, he'd take a whole *month* off, guaranteed.'

But until John's body's found, I can't relax. And neither can Jerry. He was planning more leave, but tells me he wanted to work until John 'washes up'. We're suspended in time by an unanswered question, one that isn't likely to be answered by the police, who are no longer searching. And the thought of John drifting out there all alone, or trapped under the rock-shelf, is truly unbearable. Like Jerry, I come to work to make myself feel like I'm ready to respond in case John is found.

Jerry chuckles and says, 'Lisa at St Vinnies reckons it's a hoax, that John faked his own death, took a flight to Barbados, somewhere like that, to start a new life.'

If only he'd chosen Barbados. Another if-only. I've met some survivors of suicide who've told me they didn't want to die so much as stop living the life they had, and if there'd been an alternative, like vanishing to Barbados, they might have taken that. Suicidal ideations triggered by circumstances may be an indication that we need to reinvent ourselves and start afresh.

Jerry turns on the TV. I'm curious about the different ways each paramedic in our crew has responded to John's death.

Some remain off-duty. Others, like Jerry and me, are back on the lounge John used to lie on, with his uniform shirt untucked and his rescue boots abandoned on the carpet.

As we head out on a job Jerry turns up the radio. It's *Love Song Dedications* with Richard Mercer on MIX 106.5, the soundtrack to our night shifts. John was a big fan of *Love Song Dedications*, until he broke up with Antonio. Listening to other people's love stories isn't much fun when your own is in turmoil. One caller who dedicated the *Titanic* theme song to her lover in jail was moving, I remember. But another who announced to his girlfriend and the country that, 'If you drop a tear in the ocean, when you find it again, that's when I'll stop loving you' was just too much for John. He slapped the radio like the thing had insulted him, then swore and changed the channel with a jab of his finger.

While most of the city is turning in for the night, someone's having a bad trip in a Bondi backstreet. Policemen are piled on top of a he-man who thrashes about in a drug-induced state. A small crowd of onlookers gathers on the footpath, some in pyjamas, to watch the entertainment. When I get out of the ambulance a policeman says, 'Datura.'

The plant *Datura stramonium* grows in abundance around the eastern suburbs. There's a datura tree in the lane behind my terrace. Its flowers hang like soft pink bells from its branches, but the flower's beauty is deceptive; those in the know refer to them as 'devil's trumpets'. To achieve the hallucinogenic effects of datura, some people boil the flowers down and drink the potion, while others smoke the leaves or swallow its seeds. Whatever the mode of consumption, datura is a gamble. Unlike with psilocybin mushrooms, a happy trip is not the norm and no one ever gets off lightly. An experienced user of hallucinogens once described datura to me as 'a journey for life'. He took it twelve years earlier, mixed it into a cup of Milo, and was still in recovery. The handful of datura overdoses I've encountered all presented in a similar way: bloodcurdling screams, eyes wide with horror and violent struggles.

'I can't see! I'm blind. I'm blind!' shrieks the man. One of datura's side effects is temporary blindness, as profound pupil dilation paralyses the eyes.

No wonder there are six cops holding him down.

'He was all over the road,' says the cop. 'Lashing out in a panic. No one could touch him. Nearly got hit by a car.'

We get some help to sedate the man, put him in padded restraints that attach to his wrists and his ankles, and take him to hospital. One of the cops gets in the front passenger seat and tells me that most of the police there came down from The Gap.

'Another one over, a few hours back. Found a pair of slippers, velvet ones. There was nothing in the water, nothing on the rocks. Been a few this week, eh? Crazy times.'

*

Less than a kilometre up the road from the hospital, in Potts Point, a woman has tumbled off her balcony. We've heard a few ambulances responding to falls already tonight. Two men in Coogee off a cliff by accident, and a drunk man off an overpass on the north side of town. Ever since John went over The Gap, the word 'fall' has made me feel sick. It makes me wonder what John must have felt with gravity wrenching him down. Was he looking at the disappearing railing above, the headland cliffs, the sky behind? Or was he facing the rocky shallows rushing towards him?

Jerry guesses what I'm thinking. 'We'll be okay, we don't know this lady,' he says, flicking on the siren and pushing through an intersection.

He's right. We don't know this lady. The thought should make things easier, yet I'm seeing John in all my patients and it changes how I am with them. Lots of paramedics work this way, imagining their patients are their parents, their children. To me, compassion comes without the need to superimpose the ones I cherish onto my patients. But I see how this helps to deepen the quality of care, and I know I'm doing it now with the image of John.

The woman is lying on the concrete path under her third-floor balcony. She's only semiconscious but manages to tell us she locked herself out and was scaling the wall to her balcony when she fell. Her pelvis has snapped, we're sure of it, and one of her legs sticks out at an angle, her tibia protruding through the skin. I think of the photo that the tourist took of John on the rocks. His body seemed intact, Trevor said, and he looked surprisingly peaceful, as though he were asleep. At least there is *that* to keep hold of.

There's a police cage truck in the emergency car park at St Vincent's; a couple of cops lean on the bonnet, eating ice creams in the dark. An angry guy in the back of their wagon is kicking and yelling at the top of his voice, 'She fucken infected me! I went down on her and now my lips are fucken killing! I'm gunna stab that bitch when I get outta here!'

Having seen me scrubbing blood off my stretcher, one of the officers comes over and says, 'You're mates with that ambo at Bondi who topped himself, right?'

He must be the insensitive constable who delivered the flowers, I think, and let out a sigh.

'Yeah,' I reply. 'What's up?'

'Can you take an exhibit?'

'An exhibit?'

'The guy's wallet.'

I want to say, *John, his fucking name was John, you moron.* But I let him off the hook. He's young.

'Yeah, I'll take it,' I reply.

The cop hands me a plastic bag with John's service wallet in it. I take it out and feel its weight. The leather is cracked and heavily worn. I open it up and look at his badge, a gold crest that is not so gold anymore; the gold has rubbed off almost down to the metal. It doesn't even glint when I turn it to the light. Opposite the badge is a service identity card that expired in 1998. Typical John, I think, never bothering to update his ID. In the picture he has youthful good looks, and is tanned and smiling, with an elegant moustache.

'Sign here,' says the constable, handing me a clipboard and pen, 'to confirm you've received the exhibit.'

I take the pen and sign the form.

'Love to stay and chat,' says the constable, 'but my partner's got my ice cream and it's melting.'

I laugh politely as he walks away.

When Jerry returns to the ambulance I show him the wallet and he also looks at John's mugshot for quite a while. He smiles as happy memories flood back.

'John, John, John,' he says, shaking his head. 'Life goes on after you're dead, mate. You *knew* that. People don't stop for long, they don't change much. Most people will forget about you, never think of you again. Shame, damn shame, damn waste.'

'I don't think I'll forget,' I say.

'Me neither,' says Jerry.

His family won't either, that's for sure.

'Do you think I should keep the wallet as a memory? Do you think John would mind?'

'Of course he wouldn't mind. Keep it.'

CHAPTER 17

All hope that John will be washed ashore has well and truly faded now. His memorial service will be held on the Central Coast, where his parents live, at the Catholic church they belong to. In the absence of a body, his family have decided not to call the service a funeral.

The day of the memorial is scorching hot. I planned to go alone, but Kaspia phoned and insisted on coming with me. I pick her up in Balmain and soon we're on the F3 heading up the coast together. I tell her how the other paramedics at Bondi and I noticed John deteriorating in the month before his death, beset by the guilt about his nephew, the distress about his breakup with Antonio, the despair over moving out.

'Sometimes it's only when you physically separate that you realise how connected you were, how in love . . .' I say. I don't turn to look at her when I say this, just keep my eyes on the road. I feel her staring at me in quiet thought and I start to worry that maybe she thinks the opposite, that when you physically move apart you realise how far *out* of love you've fallen.

After a minute or two of silence she gently puts her hand on mine where it's resting on the bench seat. I can't be sure if she's doing this out of sympathy because of John, or if it's something more.

The car park outside the chapel is full when we arrive; there are minibuses of paramedics who have driven up from Sydney. It's a phenomenal turnout. Several hundred ambos from all over the state are gathered together, most of them in dress uniforms with pressed white shirts, ties and medals. I could've worn my medal too, dug it out of my underwear drawer. But I know how John disliked the pomp and vanity of heroes.

We meet Jerry and Matt and all sit together. I see John's family up front, then Donna, Barry, Frank and Tracy. A slideshow tribute to John is projected on a screen. There are rolling images of him as a happy boy playing around a backyard sprinkler, others from his teenage years in which he wears neon-yellow shorts and later, in his twenties, laughing with friends in Aloha shirts. He was always a man of charisma and style, the life of the party.

I'm not surprised the Catholic priest who leads the service doesn't mention suicide. Instead he tells us John was 'lost at sea'. I'm disappointed he's skirting round the issue, but perhaps it's the metaphor that he's going for. John *was* lost at sea in his final days on earth, and I was one of the sea-going vessels that never picked him up. It's possible John would have liked the romance of being lost at sea, an image that conjures up castaways and pirates.

While most of us manage to hold ourselves together, when John's teenage niece sings 'Amazing Grace' in the most angelic of voices, people surrender. At the end of the service, all the paramedics in the church form a guard of honour at the door. Traditionally a military custom, it has long been part of what emergency workers do at the funerals of their fallen. So we stand side by side without saying a word, a passage between us for the mourners to walk through.

The melody of 'Over the Rainbow' rings out from the church as I'm shoulder to shoulder with my fellow paramedics. And I'm overcome, as many of us are, by the deepest of sadness. It's a sadness not only for John, but for all those who could see no other way than to take their own lives. It's a sadness for my guitar teacher Paul, and Martin with the John Lennon glasses, and the man called Stephen who survived his fall, and for Courtney, who cheated on her husband. I'm sad for the girl whose father John and I saw reading her suicide note at The Gap, and the hundreds of others who disappeared before we could reach them, the dozens who've died just this summer.

Face to face with my colleagues, I watch as their tears flow freely down their faces, gushing from under their sunglasses and spilling onto uniform shirts. I see their tears as they see my own. And none of us lifts a hand to wipe our faces. No one is remotely concerned about keeping that hardened composure the public assume we rely on. Our grief pours out and all of us allow it to. It's as if, in this moment, we face our own fragility, a reminder that all of us are only human, as vulnerable to loss and sorrow as any of our patients.

Out of the church and through the corridor of paramedics come John's parents and sisters. His mother is sobbing and unsteady on her feet, held upright by his elderly father. As they bravely walk they look at us and see the love we had for their son. Perhaps for the first time they truly grasp how respected and adored he was, how we stand in solidarity with him. His mother's knees give out. Two paramedics step forward to support her. Following behind her and John's father come the rest of his family, Antonio and his friends, weeping as they pass through our silent guard of honour.

Tea and biscuits are served in a nearby hall. I meet John's parents and tell them how beloved he was. Then I go and embrace Antonio and tell him how sorry I am. After that I stand around with my fellow paramedics, swapping stories of days and nights working with John. We all agree on how enjoyable it was, how funny and outrageous he could be, and the fine rapport he had with patients. Half an hour later everyone starts leaving.

It feels as if John's life is done and dusted, wrapped up and put away. But there are patients out there who still remember him, and always will. For many, calling an ambulance is sparked by a once-in-a-lifetime crisis. That day when they were critically sick or injured, that moment of drama into which John arrived to ease their anxiety or pain, is not easily forgotten. I wonder, as Kaspia drives us back to Sydney, how many patients and their friends and relatives will forever think of John. In their memories he'll live on, just as he will in ours. And what we should remember is not the way he took his life, but the way he lived it. With gentleness, humour and compassion.

On the morning of my first day back at work after the service I drag myself reluctantly up the stairs of the station, wondering if I really want this career anymore. I open John's locker and look at his stuff: a uniform shirt, two pairs of trousers, gold buttons enamelled with Maltese crosses. There's a can of deodorant and a toothbrush and toothpaste. These are simple, commonplace things that remind me how John was just like the rest of us. If pushed to a point of total despair, any of us could suffer like him, perhaps react as he did, just as I almost had. We're no strangers to death, paramedics. If we feared death we couldn't do what we do, yet our job is to keep it at bay.

★

With coffees in hand, Matt and I sit in the ambulance in the car park at the beach. It's sweltering outside, and our aircon hums. Out at sea, black clouds loom on the horizon and lightning flickers. Neither of us is in much of a mood for our usual jokey banter. We sip our coffees without a word and know perfectly well what the other is thinking about.

Then, as if delivered from above, a remarkable thing happens.

A man has collapsed at a restaurant in Double Bay and no one's quite sure if he's breathing or not. We're told he's making gurgling sounds. He's in his eighties, and I'm cynical as ever about his chances, but Matt and I still make an effort. Matt drives hard, our tyres screech round corners. He gets from Bondi to Double Bay in less than three minutes. I sling my stethoscope round my neck and pull on some gloves.

We turn into Bay Street and see a man vigorously pumping on the chest of our patient, who is on the footpath, splayed awkwardly between café tables.

Matt cuts the siren. I step out of the ambulance and slide open the side door in one fluid motion, grabbing oxygen and the Lifepak defibrillator. I ask a waitress to shift furniture out of the way and several bystanders rush to help her make room. The man doing CPR has muscular arms, and performs the best compressions I've seen. The patient's chest has a 'zipper' down the middle: an old scar from a bypass.

'Keep going, mate,' I tell the first-aider. 'Good work.'

Matt attaches the pads and charges the Lifepak. Meanwhile I slip an airway between the man's teeth, place a mask on his face and begin ventilations. Matt's ready to shock.

'Here we go,' he says, then calls, 'Everyone clear!'

The man doing CPR lifts his hands off the chest and we check it's a shockable rhythm. Matt pushes the button and the patient's body contracts in a spasm then relaxes again. It's a little confronting for people to see, and the bystanders gasp. I ask the man who had been doing compressions to continue CPR, noticing how drenched in sweat he's become. He won't be needing the gym today.

After another two minutes of CPR, once we've charged the machine and go for another shock, I see a regular rhythm appear on the screen. I feel for a pulse.

'Is that what I think it is?' asks Matt, looking up.

We confirm at the femoral artery. Yes, the man has a pulse. We haven't even got an IV or given him adrenalin. Just CPR and a shock and he's back.

We've saved a life.

People can see the surprise on our faces.

'I can't believe it,' I exclaim, as Matt congratulates the man who did compressions.

The patient's son arrives on scene and tells us his father had his first bypass twenty years ago. He's hardly a picture of health, and I remind myself not to get too hopeful about his return of circulation. The man hasn't woken yet and it's likely he won't. Despite getting excellent CPR from the time of collapse, in all likelihood he'll have brain damage from lack of oxygen. He's not the first cardiac-arrest patient to get their pulse back but never come to. It's the usual scenario.

When our backup crew arrives, we roll the old man onto a spine board and lift him onto our stretcher. It's only a two-minute trip to hospital and we offload at St Vincent's straight into the resus bay. Doctors and nurses swarm around us.

'Well done,' says a cardiologist, patting me on the back.

Outside, I shake hands with Matt.

'This could be the one,' I say.

'If it is, it'll be my first too,' he replies.

Both of us are beaming.

'Funny, isn't it. Twelve years in the job and no save, then just after John dies, this guy . . .'

It seems to me like divine encouragement, or perhaps John's gift from the afterlife.

The man's name was George. A couple of days later, after night shift, I visit him in the intensive-care ward. When I pull back the curtain he's sitting in a recliner having breakfast, sipping on tea. He looks so carefree and comfortable, as if his hospital stay is a little getaway.

'I nearly died, you say?' He slurps on his tea.

'Yes, your heart stopped.'

'Oh dear. You don't mind passing me that toast there, do you?'

I pass him his toast and know there's no way I can make him comprehend how exceptional his survival is. Before waking up in ICU the last thing George remembers was drinking an espresso in Double Bay while discussing the business of his hotel chain with a friend.

George speaks in a muffled tone, a bit like Marlon Brando in *The Godfather*. He smiles and says, 'When I get out, I'll take you and your partner to lunch at one of my hotels, okay?'

His offer of a posh lunch makes me less annoyed at him for his laissez-faire attitude about his heart attack. I'm disappointed when he never follows through with his invitation, but I suppose for George his cardiac arrest was just another medical inconvenience. Why should he care that I've waited my career to save his life?

On my way out I see the doctor looking after George. I've met her before, down in Emergency. Her eyes light up and she asks if I was the one who brought him in. Yeah, I say, my partner and me. The guy doing CPR at the scene was crucial too. Then I tell her this was my first real save in twelve years, as far as I know. But she doesn't believe me. She's been fully qualified for only eighteen months and saved dozens of patients already. I remind her that the ones who collapse in a hospital have a much better chance of survival, as medical staff are on hand to help. Many who drop in the street or at home don't get CPR at all. By the time an ambulance arrives ten minutes later, their chances are poor. The doctor shakes her head. I can tell she feels pity for me.

'Thanks to George I can happily retire now, right?'

She laughs, and says, 'Or it'll buy you another twelve years in the job.'

'I don't think I can wait twelve years for another save, doc.'

She frowns. 'There are many ways to save a life. You know that, right?'

I leave the hospital, and before going home to bed I make a special trip to The Gap. Last time I was here, just after John went over, we didn't have time to reflect much. We were picking up Veronica, the girl who denied she was planning to die.

The spot where I saw the flowers that day is easy to find because another paramedic has put a cross on the railing and secured it there with medical tape. The flowers are looking worse for wear, though there's a fresh bunch cable-tied to the fence a metre away. Up here one can never be sure who the flowers are for. At least two more souls have left from this spot since John went over.

As I look down into the mouth of The Gap the waves rush across the rock-shelf, then draw back again. This would have been the level of tide when John took his life. It's rare that I come here in my own time, and it really is a beautiful place. How many people intent on dying are seduced by this beauty and decide to live instead? How many come up here with death in mind, then quietly walk away? Beauty should stimulate happiness, admiration, gratitude, joy. Perhaps John and the many others go over too quickly for the beauty to work. Or maybe they're just blinded by despair.

I think about the parting words of the ICU doctor. *There are many ways to save a life.* Why am I so obsessed with cardiac arrests, trying to save patients with the poorest prognosis, basing my value as a medic on those outcomes? I may have an unlucky track record in that respect but like many paramedics, I've talked a lot of people down from the edge, convinced them not to take their lives. I hold that thought and let it grow, then I turn my back on The Gap and head to the car.

CHAPTER 18

It's already thirty degrees at 9 am, when Jerry and I drive down to North Bondi and park beside the Mr Whippy van. We unzip our rescue boots and go to the water's edge, roll up the bottom of our uniform pants and dip our toes in the shallows. Together we inspect little rock pools that shimmer in the sun like odd-shaped mirrors. When my shadow passes over one I can see it's filled with waving seaweed and red anemones. Jerry's close behind me and I hear the crackling of the portable radio that he's carrying, a necessity so unnatural and distracting.

'Jerry!' I call out, beckoning him over, showing him the rock pool.

'Sea enemies,' observes Jerry matter-of-factly, reaching a hand into the water and sticking his forefinger into the tiny mouth of a hungry anemone. It puckers up on his fingertip just as the portable radio splutters and breaks the tranquillity again.

Sydney, 402? Exact location, please . . .

With one finger in a sea anemone and another on the press-to-talk button, Jerry answers that we are beachside and available to respond.

'Copy,' comes the controller. 'Female unwell, up the road from you.'

At the back of the ambulance we dry off our feet with hospital towels. Working with Jerry is not too different to working with John. How much fun John had with us down here at Bondi for all those years. How much more he could have had.

As we drive to the job I turn to Jerry and say, 'I wonder where John is right now. You ever wonder that?'

'Belly of a whale?' replies Jerry. 'I don't know. It's not him, it's his body. It's not like we'll get a living John back again. Think about it. He'd probably want his ashes scattered out at sea, anyway. He loved the ocean.'

People need answers, I tell him. They need closure.

Jerry looks annoyed. 'Closure is bullshit. People need acceptance, so they can live with what's happened.'

As we enter the house of the elderly woman we've been sent to, I notice what looks like a retro child's bedroom.

The colour scheme is brown and orange, and there's a lava lamp and an Evel Knievel figurine on the chest of drawers. A Snoopy poster hangs on the wall above the bed. When I ask the woman about the room she tells us that her five-year-old son, her only child, was hit by a car and killed in 1975. She hasn't moved a thing in his bedroom since that day, just vacuumed and dusted it every so often.

For a tragedy like this, closure might be impossible. But acceptance is almost as futile.

We hear the news after lunchtime: Heath Ledger has died in his Manhattan apartment. The bulletin is announced on the radio as we're driving less than a kilometre from Heath's former mansion overlooking Bronte.

'Unbelievable,' says Jerry.

'Unbelievable,' I repeat.

'John and Heath in the same month.'

'Too weird.'

'I wonder if they're finally hanging out in the afterlife. It's what John always wanted, wasn't it?'

On the North Bondi headland, a stone's throw from the ambulance station, a man is standing on the edge, high above the sea. We arrive before the police, and walk to the crest of the hill. A young boy meets us and says we should hurry, the man's barely holding on.

'You're treating,' says Jerry, dropping the kits and pushing me forward.

The girl we took off The Gap the night after John fell was already in custody. But this man is dressed in black, his shoes are off, and he's over the edge, standing on a ledge, holding on with one hand. I approach him slowly and can see his body is drenched in sweat.

'Hi there,' I say from a distance, then introduce myself when I'm a few metres closer. He yells, 'Get away! I'm gunna do it! I don't want your help!'

There's no fence up here, and I creep forward a little and sit down on the clifftop.

I repeat my name and ask him for his. 'I just want to sit with you, please,' I say.

He turns back to look at the sea surging against the crags far below, and it seems to me he's shifting his weight. His body language tells me he has every intention of following through. I've no doubt that if the boy hadn't found him, and if we hadn't arrived so quickly, we'd be dealing with a body on the rocks like John.

'I really want to talk with you,' I say.

'Why do you care? No one gives a shit!'

'Believe it or not, I *do* care.'

'You're only doing your job.'

Our conversation feels like movie dialogue. Plenty of conversations we have in this line of work could be lifted from an action-film screenplay. I've always wondered to what extent fictional drama informs off-screen behaviour: life imitating art, as they say.

'Seriously, mate, it would've been easier for me to wait for the police and let *them* talk to you. But I'm here because I care. I don't want you to do this.'

After thinking for a second he says, 'My name's Michael.'

'Thanks, Michael. Any chance you can come up and away from the edge? You're making me nervous. Better we chat away from the edge.'

'The sea is calling me, mate. It's calling. I've driven down from Queensland for this. I've planned it for months. I'm going over, I'm telling you straight, I'm telling you now. There's nothing you can do about it. You don't understand. No one gives a shit.'

'Surely there's someone out there you mean something to. What about parents? Are your parents still alive?'

'I was fucking adopted. My parents threw me to the dogs. And my adoptive parents abused me. They tied me up. They beat me. My adopted father sexually abused me, he raped me. Do you know how that feels? As a child? The people you're meant to trust, the ones who you rely on for your needs, the ones who are meant to show you love, abusing you? Beating you and making you do fucked-up shit?'

I shake my head. I can't reply.

Michael is trembling, he's in the grip of anger. 'No, you don't know how it feels, do you. I've got no one, mate. I've got no family. I've got no friends. I've got no job. I've got nothing.'

'What about a partner, Michael?'

'Partner? Yeah, I had a partner if you want to know. She fucked my best friend and pissed off with him. And when she pissed off she took all my shit. She was everything I had. Finally I thought I'd found a person I could trust, because I didn't even know the word "trust" existed. Understand? Then she fucked off.'

'Is there anything at all that makes you happy?' I ask, clutching at straws.

'Happy? What the fuck is happy? You know what makes me happy is to look down and see those waves calling my name. You know what it's like to live with schizophrenia? To feel worthless? Every moment of every day I hear my adoptive father telling me I'm dirty and worthless. He's right here in my head. *Fucking worthless piece of shit*, he says. Do you know what it's like to hear yourself being called a fucking worthless piece of shit every waking second of your life? It's a voice you can't escape. My whole life has been fucked up from the word go. Death can't be any worse, can it? When life is hell, death looks pretty good.'

For perhaps the first time in a situation like this, I find I'm lost for words. Jerry and the others often make me do the talk-downs because they know I like counselling, and my track record's good. But now I'm stuck, and it's because I feel unqualified. Not in the professional sense, but in life experience. I'm a man with a healthy body and mind, raised in a middle-class family, with generous, loving parents. I have loyal friends, a nice home and a beautiful partner who I feel I'm slowly reconciling with. As Michael tells me about all the things he doesn't have to live for, I think about the things I do have. Who am I to talk him down? What if I had walked in *his* shoes? Wouldn't I be standing there too, at the edge of the cliff? How arrogant I am to tell him how great life is or how much better it can get. For all his life, Michael's hoped for things to get better. But they haven't, and now he's here, at the end of the road, an escape from his hell.

A feeling of mercy silences me. It makes me want to walk away and let him go. But then I think, what if all my blessings were precisely for moments like these? What if my job is to pass on the love I've been given?

Behind me, about twenty metres back, a group of cops are chatting with Jerry. There's a police inspector too, and an ambulance commander in a dress shirt and tie. They've allowed me the space that I need, trusting I've built a rapport with the patient, not wanting to interrupt, hoping that sooner rather than later I can bring the guy in. From the way Jerry's glancing anxiously over I can tell he's praying that I don't mess this up.

'Just let me do this, mate,' pleads Michael with tears on his face. 'I want to go. If you really want to save me, then save me from my fucked-up life by letting me go to the waves.'

He turns his back on me and I sense he's about to release his grip. I get a hit of adrenalin, my stomach churns, my carotid pulse pounds. If I make a grab for him, I'll go over too. He's too big, too heavy, and I'm not in a harness connected to ropes. Words are all I have. And I don't care if I sound 'a little bit Oprah'. Life is precious and I believe in transformation, in the promise of healing.

'Michael, stop. Please. You're in a dark place, I hear you. Don't lose hope. It's hard for you to see right now, but there's always hope. Things can turn around for people, I've seen it. People can be reborn, start over. People like you. You're not *meant* to die. I don't believe that. If this moment is fate, then so is me being here with you, talking to you. Don't you think that's a sign? Don't you think it's fate that I've met you, and you've met me? You think the waves are calling you, but I'm calling you louder. Come back from the edge, Michael, please.'

Then I mention John, and I know it won't be the last time I do. 'A good friend of mine went over these cliffs, further up, at The Gap. It happened last month. His name was John. He was a paramedic like me. I know he didn't have the pain you have. But he had enough pain to end it. And that's what he did. We loved him very much and all of us are grieving.

We really are. We loved him and we miss him. We all wish he hadn't done it because we honestly believe that life could've improved for him. Just as I believe life can get better for you. I know you don't think this can happen. You have no reason to believe that it can. But one day the reward for your courage to survive will be happiness, and you'll know it when you find it. I wish I was given the chance to convince my friend John of that before he died, to remind him of the beauty in this world. Unfortunately, I never had that chance. But I *do* have that chance with you, right now. Take my hand, Michael. Turn around and take the hand I'm holding out to you.'

I don't expect him to, but he turns around slowly and grasps my hand and pulls himself up. Then he has his arms around me and is sobbing into my shoulder, sobbing like a child. I hold him and let him weep. Somewhere in my mind I hear John laughing ever so gently with a twinkle in his eye, saying, 'Honestly, do you really have to hug them?' And I smile to myself.

As I lead Michael down the slope of the golf course Jerry is beside me and a dozen cops behind, everyone walking silently to the ambulance. My hand is on Michael's shoulder as he plods along with his head stooped low, crying quietly.

After putting Michael in the ambulance, I step out for a quick word with the ambulance commander.

'You okay?' he asks me.

'Thanks, I'm fine.'

He shakes my hand. 'Congratulations, mate. A job well done. Listen, I'm going to put you forward for a service citation.'

'A what?' I ask.

'Citation. Bravery award.'

'For what?'

'Saving this bloke.'

A sigh escapes me. 'With all due respect, sir, I don't want a citation.'

My supervisor looks confused, but I have nothing more to say. I get into the ambulance and slam the side door shut behind me, then take a seat with my patient, Michael. I call out to Jerry in the front, 'Right to go, mate!'

And he pulls away towards the hospital, making sure to take the scenic route past the beach.

In memory of
John Vincent Dixon
7/11/1962 – 10/1/2008

MENTAL HEALTH SUPPORT SERVICES

Adult

Lifeline: 13 11 14
lifeline.org.au

Suicide Call Back Service: 1300 659 467
suicidecallbackservice.org.au

Beyond Blue: 1300 24 636
beyondblue.org.au

MensLine Australia: 1300 789 987
mensline.org.au

Youth

Kids Helpline: 1800 551 800
kidshelpline.com.au

headspace: 1800 650 890
headspace.org.au

ReachOut: au.reachout.com

Other resources

Life in Mind (suicide prevention portal):
lifeinmindaustralia.com.au

Head to Health (mental health portal):
headtohealth.gov.au

SANE (online forums): sane.org

Further reading

'Answering the Call: A survey on the mental health and well-being of police and emergency service workers in Australia' (Beyond Blue, 2018)